Nervous Breakdown

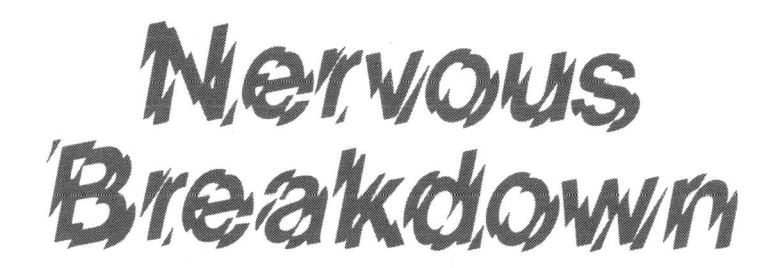

Nervous Breakdown

What is it?
What causes it?
Who can help?

Jenny Cozens

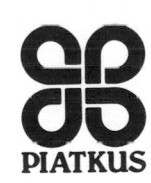

PIATKUS

To Ian

© 1988 Jenny Cozens

First published in 1988 by
Judy Piatkus (Publishers) Limited
5 Windmill Street, London W1P 1HF

Reprinted in 1993

The moral right of the author has been asserted

A catalogue record for this title is available from the British Library

ISBN 0–7499–1204–9

Cover design by Jennie Smith

Phototypeset in 10/12 Linotron Baskerville by
Phoenix Photosetting, Chatham
Printed and bound in Great Britain by
Mackays of Chatham PLC, Chatham, Kent

Contents

Acknowledgements

I would like to thank all the psychologists and psychiatrists who, as colleagues, have offered their different perspectives over the years, and to my fellow researchers at the MRC/ESRC Social and Applied Psychology Unit in Sheffield who have helped me acquire a critical eye on research.

Specifically I am indebted to Dr Michael Barkham and Ms Gillian Hardy for their readings of early chapters, to Dr Stephen Blomfield, for providing invaluable comments from a psychiatric perspective, and to Ms Kathryn Beadsley for her patient preparation of the manuscript.

Finally my thanks to all my clients over the years who have had the courage to share their troubles and who have taught me so much.

Part One

Chapter

1

What do you mean by a nervous breakdown?

When I was young it was my teachers or my mother's friends who had nervous breakdowns. People talked about them in whispers, but with a wise look and a sympathetic tone. The image I had was of nerves – long thin white messenger systems running throughout their bodies – stopping working in some way. Becoming sore or swollen, or dying at the ends; shredding or, stretched to breaking point, finally snapping. Any definition seemed impossible, since the term appeared to be used so widely. At one end there was Miss Smith, our German teacher, standing in front of us with tears in her eyes, screwing her handkerchief round and round, both angry and upset and then absent for a fortnight. When she returned, bright and cheerful, she'd announced she was leaving at the end of the term to be an air hostess.

At the other end of the spectrum was Mr Johnson, our neighbour, who'd 'gone away' for nine months or more and now sat gazing blankly just above the fence, hardly speaking to his family and ignoring me completely. The only information I could come across upon the subject I found in books illustrated with pictures of the horrors of Victorian asylums and early treatments, which filled me with a secret unmentionable fear that I too could become mad and end up somewhere like that, a fear I now know is very common but almost never shared with others.

Later, as I trained as a clinical psychologist, I came into contact with people suffering at all points on the spectrum and my fear dissolved as my knowledge grew. The term 'nervous breakdown' was never used in the professional groups I mixed with; instead people were described as depressed or anxious or suffering from anorexia nervosa or schizophrenia. But still, when someone comes for help, having poured out their problems and their anguish and their confusion, they will ask, 'Am I having a nervous breakdown?' They may add: 'Of course, I don't really know what a nervous breakdown is. I thought I did, but now I'm wondering if this is what's happening to me.' And I know that very often they're scared stiff they're going mad.

This is an area where mystery adds nothing: the lack of knowledge that mystery involves feeds fear, and fear is the basis of many psychological problems that come under the umbrella term, 'nervous breakdown'. My aim in this book is to take away the mystery – to talk about the range of problems which mean that your life has broken down in some way, that it has changed for the worse, not because of any physical disability, but because of the very real pressures that exist for many of you, or because the way you see life, or aspects of it, or the way you see yourself has changed. It discusses what you should look for as signs that things are going wrong and describes the variety of help that is available. I've illustrated this with the stories of people I know, with details changed to protect their anonymity. Some of you will use the descriptions and the stories to decide that you have no psychological problems that need help; some will perhaps recognise aspects of yourselves or of people close to you and decide that it's time to see what can be done. Others of you will already know there is a problem and use this book to learn more about it and the ways it can be eased.

The term 'breakdown', with its links to machinery and cars, has its problems. It implies something mechanical about us as human beings, something that an expert can tinker with – knowing exactly where to put his or her spanner – and get back on to the road again. In fact, as this book will show throughout, we are all extremely complex individuals, each unique and each subject to a variety of pressures both from within and without. In this sense any mechanical analogy fails completely to represent the human condition. Nevertheless, many people find the term 'breakdown' useful, giving them an understandable view of what happens, providing a rationale for regular maintenance and care, both internally and externally, and also implying that what breaks down can be mended. A psychologist I know found his telephone number was only one digit different to that of the Automobile Association. Few days would go by without someone phoning him and asking for help with a breakdown. So close is the comparison between the human and the car in this respect, that it was often some way into the conversation before he would realise that the problem was purely mechanical!

The dictionary defines breakdown as a collapse or stoppage. 'Collapse' implies a sudden, swift deterioration, a total breaking apart of the structures that hold people together and make them who they are. In the analogy of the car, it is the blowing up of the engine, or the failure of the brakes or the steering, that instantly stops the driver and the machine interacting in the usual way. In the person, it is this dramatic type of change that most of us think of as a breakdown, easily recognisable, sometimes bizarre, something that puts the person out of reach and out of reason to those around. These are often called **psychotic** breakdowns and are seen by some to be qualitatively different to normal behaviour – not part of a continuum with normality, but something else. Essentially, these are the behaviours that people label mad.

A stoppage, however, implies something slower; something that builds up over time. Again using the car as an analogy, it may be the building up of carbon on the spark plugs which makes the engine falter at red lights so the driver learns to keep the choke out just a little; or the gradual wearing down of the clutch which makes him rev the engine more each time he starts. These things, happening over time, allow the car to go on being driven while the driver adjusts his or her actions gradually as things slowly deteriorate. Eventually the car will collapse and stop, and when it has been mended the driver will wonder at the change that has occurred and realise, looking back, just how bad things had been for some time. In humans such a breakdown will also be much less obvious than the speedy dramatic kind. The changes may be so slow that neither those suffering nor the people who are close to them will necessarily recognise, at least at first, that things are going wrong. Since both of you will adjust your behaviour, it may be some time before you realise that the interactions between you have changed and are becoming problematic.

These changes, which all cause some form of distress, are often called **neurotic** disorders by the medical profession, a term which implies that they are on a continuum with normal feelings and behaviours – we all experience them to some degree or other. Whether the change is fast or slow, whether the behaviour or the emotions are simply exaggerations of behaviours or emotions that we all experience, or whether they are quite different and bizarre, the point of breakdown is the point at which it's recognised that things are out of control.

This book then should help you to recognise the signs and symptoms that suggest that you, or someone else, might be heading towards breakdown, so that perhaps you will be better able to judge that help is necessary, and to become more aware of what is available.

There are areas which are sometimes confused with nervous breakdowns and which are not dealt with in this book. For example, although people with a mental handicap may suffer from psychological problems, just like those of us with more obvious abilities, they may equally well be perfectly happy and relaxed. Their disabilities come from damage to their brain, often at or before birth, and the services provided for them are quite separate and different to those discussed in this book.

Also, apart from some discussion of the dementias in Chapter 12, I'm not discussing problems that occur from actual physical changes in the brain; for example those that may come about from head injuries or tumours.

Wide blanket terms like 'nervous breakdown' or 'psychological problems' have their benefits and their disadvantages. The benefits come from the fact that while they remain uncategorised into conditions or diagnoses, such as depression or phobias or schizophrenia, we can approach them with a more open mind, taking the problems of each person as something unique to him or her. This doesn't mean we don't recognise patterns of problems that we've met before, which makes it useful in knowing what to do to help, but it means we don't become rigid in our knowledge or our treatments. This is especially important with psychological problems or 'mental illness', since all the conditions in fact overlap considerably and research shows that precise diagnosis is often very difficult. So someone who is anxious will often become depressed as well; someone who is depressed may become dependent on alcohol; someone who is obsessional will inevitably suffer from anxiety, and so on. This approach is psychological rather than medical, where the problems are largely seen as illnesses and, as such, able to be categorised into diagnoses.

The other difficulty with diagnosis is that treating the problems as illnesses which are medically defined implies that something has happened to the individual almost from the outside, and that much of the responsibility for cure will also come from there. When you do suffer a nervous breakdown, though drugs and other treatment will often help, it may be far more important to recognise that you and those around you need to change yourselves or your surroundings in some way. Sometimes you can help yourself to do this and often you will be given guidance where it's needed, but no one can do the actual changing except you. Hence the Californian joke which asks: 'How many psychoanalysts does it take to change a light bulb?' Answer: 'One, but the light bulb's really got to want to change!'

Moreover, thoughts about 'mental illness' alter over time. Unlike physical illnesses, no one is able to look through the microscope and see the picture of manic-depression or any other condition. What's 'normal' and 'abnormal' can only be socially defined. Someone who hears God talking to her, like Joan of Arc, would today be likely to be diagnosed as schizophrenic; on the other hand, homosexuality was not so long ago thought of as mental illness, whereas today of course it's not. Alcohol addiction too comes on and off the list of diagnoses as views about it change with new knowledge or opinion.

There is a more fundamental criticism of the idea that these problems are mental illnesses. This has been made by Professor David Smail from Nottingham who points out that to see them as illnesses takes the blame away from the social conditions, not just of poverty, but also of the fantasy world of consumerism which makes us always less than the media ideal. But whether psychological problems are classifiable as mental illnesses or not is an argument that will keep those involved debating for many years to come. The important thing to remember is that there are very valid arguments against thinking of them as distinct illnesses and to keep these in mind when seeking help. About one woman in six and one man in nine will ask for help for their distress and most of these at some stage will consult a doctor, whether their general practitioner or a psychiatrist. When you do consult your doctors,

7

because of their medical training, the majority of you who seek help will receive a diagnosis.

The benefit of diagnosis is that it provides a short-hand way of talking about and understanding psychological problems. It allows self-help groups and support groups to be formed who know clearly that they have something definite in common, who can join together to improve the services they receive. Moreover, calling them 'illnesses' has definitely helped to remove some of the stigma that once attached itself to these problems. However it undeniably still exists, perhaps because by labelling someone 'ill' you can ignore the fact that he or she has been treated badly by society.

More and more people who have suffered breakdowns now talk about them more openly, and some of these are in public life. John Ogdon, the pianist, has described his experiences of manic-depression; Evelyn Waugh wrote about his brief period of bizarre thoughts and behaviours in his novel *The Ordeal of Gilbert Pinfold*; Glenys Kinnock has discussed the depression she experienced after the birth of her second child, though other political figures have been less open. Stuart Sutherland, Professor of Psychology at Brighton, wrote a book called simply *Breakdown* in which he described his obsessional jealousy and eventual hospitalisation. In this he points out: 'It is as likely to affect the great, like Newton or Van Gogh, as the lowly.' He quotes Sargant, a well-known British psychiatrist, who claims that more than one British prime minister has made suicide attempts before attaining that office. Many others have suffered attacks of depression, often described in the newspapers as 'nervous exhaustion' or 'fatigue'. Sargant writes: 'To eliminate all those in high public positions in Great Britain who have had ECT would deplete our ranks of some very competent people indeed, still more so if one extended the ban to all those with a history of depression.'

Finally, it's true that, although labelling someone (for example, as having anxiety or manic-depression) causes undeniable difficulties, people often welcome a diagnosis because it narrows down their problems to something they can understand, rather than having the frightening vagueness of a term like 'nervous breakdown' and all it might imply.

For this reason, Part Two of the book is divided into chapters, many of which are named by the common diagnoses. Its path and progression, however, implies much more of a continuum, starting with stress reactions and moving on to the so-called neurotic disorders, such as depression, anxiety and obsessions, and the psychological problems related to physical conditions. These chapters aim primarily to inform you of the signs that indicate that things are going wrong and to give you some guidelines about whether self-help might be possible or what other help is available and may be offered for each specific problem.

The final chapters discuss the so-called 'psychotic' disorders, such as manic-depression and schizophrenia, and also dementia, where individuals may for a time have insufficient insight to seek help for themselves. These chapters may give extra information to those of you already suffering from these problems and also be helpful to those relatives and friends who are worried about what is happening and what they can do to help.

Although I have attempted to cover the main ideas about the causes and treatments of these problems, I am still bound to view them primarily through my experience as a clinical psychologist. Nevertheless, both psychiatrists and psychologists have given advice and information on the issues in this book, and I am very grateful for their help. In splitting the book into chapters that reflect diagnoses, I am going along with medical classification rather than the psychological approach of taking each individual and each problem as it comes. I am adopting this structure for convenience – both yours and mine – because psychological problems are so complex and classifying them in this way lets me make useful and realistic generalisations and relates too to the way you may discuss the problems with your doctor and your friends. On the other hand, please stay aware that the categories implied by the chapters are by no means watertight and in fact overlap considerably. Freud saw all psychological problems as on a continuum with normality and no one yet has shown that this is wrong.

Chapter

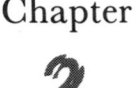

Types of help for psychological problems

The varieties of help available are discussed more specifically in each chapter, but this review of treatments will give you a better understanding of the reasons behind the therapies and the different training involved for the various mental health professionals who deliver them. You can read it now to acquaint yourself with various methods and professionals concerned, or you can use it as a reference chapter as you read the rest of the book.

The type of help which is suggested or offered to you will vary considerably according to your own knowledge and the views of your general practitioner and local psychiatric services. It depends too on where you live, since different health districts and regions of the country may provide quite radically different facilities. Research has shown that unfortunately it also varies with other factors such as which sex you are (women are more often prescribed minor tranquillisers than men, for example), what age you are and what class and race (older people and working-class people are less likely to receive psychotherapy, for example, than the younger and middle class). This is not to say that these differences are necessarily bad – behavioural therapy or drugs may be as appropriate as psychotherapy in some cases – just that treatment for psychological problems is not as clear-cut as it is for physical ones.

If you choose to go to your GP in the first place with your

problems, and he or she feels unable to treat you, you may be referred on directly to a clinical psychologist or to a psychiatrist, most of whom work in the NHS. A move towards community services means that mental health centres under the NHS are being set up in many parts of Britain, and you can usually approach these directly. Within their teams of professionals many of the treatments discussed will be available.

Basically, help can be grouped into three main areas: self-help; psychological help, such as psychotherapy or behaviour therapy; and physical treatments, which are provided only by doctors and which include drugs, electro-convulsive treatment and, extremely rarely, surgery. Hospitalisation is not actually a treatment in itself, but a place to provide treatments more easily. However, it may be seen also as an asylum, in the original sense of the word – a safe place away from the pressures of life, which may have its role to play early on in therapy.

SELF-HELP

There are many forms of self-help techniques which may be used to counteract stress and to deal with problems when they are recognisable but still feel controllable. These will be discussed in more detail in each chapter, if they are applicable, but generally include some form of relaxation, via tapes or classes or yoga, or of health promotion such as exercise, rest and reducing or eliminating things that harm you such as alcohol, cigarettes and mind-altering drugs.

The other main form of self-help comes from the support and companionship of a group who are suffering similar things to you. These groups may be organised locally, even started by yourself, or be part of some large nationwide concern. It can be an immense relief to know that you are not alone in your problems, and that other people understand so well what you have faced and what you are feeling. The only danger with these groups is that they can occasionally entail little more than the swapping of symptoms, and that you may 'need' to keep your problems in order to remain a member. If the people in the group remain your only source of support and understanding, ending your psychological difficulties may not be such an attractive outcome as staying qualified as a member of the group!

Many such groups are long established and relevant ones are listed at the end of the book. Other local ones may be obtained from your Citizens Advice Bureau or from your nearest MIND office. If you wish to begin your own group, information on ways of doing this, and of avoiding the pitfalls, can be obtained from the Women's Therapy and Counselling Service and from the Mind Your Self Project, both based in Leeds, and from the Self-Help Team based in Nottingham.

PSYCHOLOGICAL THERAPIES

These are the therapies, derived largely from psychological theory, which are non-physical, based essentially around talking, but usually involving some aspect of experiencing. For example, they may require you to experience your feelings – your anxiety, your anger, your despair – rather than shut them up and pretend they don't exist; or they may necessitate confronting your fears in the real world, as when someone stands up to a difficult parent or spouse after years of silent fuming, or pats a dog after years of terror at the thought of even meeting one.

Because so many different professions are trained in the various treatments, I'll use the general term 'therapist' to describe those who give some form of psychological help.

The opening up and experiencing of feelings is covered by the general term **psychotherapy**. The therapist aims to provide a safe environment for the client to consider the problems that brought him or her into treatment, and often, in **psychodynamic psychotherapy**, will use the relationship between the two of them as a way of experiencing and recognising the inappropriate ways that the client may relate to people outside. For example, clients may appear with a slightly hostile, aggressive manner, complaining that they have trouble dealing with people at work or at home. Over the course of therapy, they may come to realise that this manner, often pointed out in the sessions themselves, appears whenever they fear ridicule or humiliation. They may come to realise just how much of this fear belongs not to the present at all, but to humiliating experiences in childhood which they learned to protect themselves against by being the first to raise their fists or make some cutting remark. The insight gained allows people to develop more appropriate ways of relating now rather than staying stuck in the protective but limiting ways they learnt in childhood.

Sessions will usually be hourly, once or twice a week, and may continue for a year or more; with rarely fewer than a dozen sessions. Rather than involving a 'shrink' of one's mind, people find it a liberating and often a creative experience.

Another aim of psychotherapy may be to increase self-esteem by making clients feel valued and accepted, even when they reveal the parts of themselves they hate the most. This 'non-judgemental unqualified regard' forms the basis of the **client-centred approach** to therapy and counselling and was begun by the American clinical psychologist, Carl Rogers. Like other forms of psychotherapy, it rarely involves the giving of advice, but rather helps to clear away the psychological debris and provide the space you need to make decisions and to understand things better.

The general term psychotherapy also includes **psychoanalysis**, as begun by Sigmund Freud, which aims to explore the client's earliest conflicts and the ways these relate to his or her present problems. Classically it involves the client lying on a couch with the analyst out of view behind him; sessions are usually three to five times a week and may go on for a number of years. Freud's contribution to the understanding of psychological problems is enormous and still underlies most therapists' work, though Rogers' has perhaps been more influential in the method of delivery.* Fully qualified psychoanalysts are comparatively rare in Britain, especially outside London and Edinburgh.

Gestalt therapy, less commonly practised in this country than in the States, concentrates very much on the 'here-and-now' of the therapy session and aims to get clients to release and to integrate shut-off parts of their minds and bodies. They may be asked to express some statement by using their bodies, or to rid themselves of anger by talking to or shouting at an empty chair containing the imagined object of their rage. These methods have the aim of releasing considerable pent-up emotion which not only affects and limits our minds but also our bodies. Thus they have been used

---

* There is no way I can do justice to the depth and the excitement of psychoanalytic theory, but some flavour of the experience is described in Marie Cardinal's autobiographical novel, *The Words to Say It*.

successfully both with people who are depressed and also those with certain physical problems such as arthritis and back pain, which are sometimes linked with pent-up rage. Such therapies are often very brief, usually taking fewer than a dozen sessions and often take place in groups. Their methods sometimes formed part of the encounter group movement which is generally regarded as being helpful only to those who are psychologically fit and *not* for anyone suffering a breakdown.

Psychotherapy may be individual or in groups. **A therapy group** may be brought together because the individuals are suffering similar problems, or may be more mixed in terms of both problems and sexes. They are particularly useful for people suffering relationship problems, since again they presume that these will manifest themselves swiftly in the group situation. Although at first individuals feel higher levels of anxiety in groups, this is usually overcome as the group, with the help of the therapist, learns to trust and to support its members. Self-esteem is increased by being able to help the others. In hospitals groups may be 'open'; that is, people join and leave as they are admitted or discharged. In outpatient settings or in the private or charitable sector, groups are usually 'closed' with around 8–12 members and no one new entering the group once it has begun. The book which John Cleese wrote with Robin Skynner, *Families and How to Survive Them*, came out of his experiences in such a group.

Family therapy is a form of group therapy used when the relationships within the family are in some way disturbed. Often a child will be sent as 'the patient', the one who is most easily identifiable as having the problem, but the therapist may offer this therapy if he or she feels that the other family members may possibly be contributing unwittingly to the child's behaviour. Apart from general behaviour problems, it is used successfully in cases of anorexia nervosa, in incest cases, and in helping to prevent relapse in young people with schizophrenia.

Marital therapy is provided either by a single therapist or by one of each sex to balance the couple seeking help. Its aim is to open communication between you in a constructive way; to air both grievances and appreciation whether with a view to reconciliation, or so that separation, although sad, doesn't leave each partner with unfinished business that could then be taken over to spoil a future relationship. It may, if necessary, include **sex**

therapy to help you both achieve more satisfaction from that part of your relationship. Marriage Guidance Counsellors have training in both these areas, or occasionally one or both may be provided by therapists in the NHS.

The other main branch of psychological treatments is **behavioural** or **cognitive-behavioural therapy**. **Behaviour therapy** comes from experimental psychology's learning theory. It has shown that behaviours, both appropriate and inappropriate, are learned and so can be un-learned. Thus someone who has learned to fear spiders may learn to approach them unafraid, and the therapy sessions are aimed to bring this about, probably by learning to associate relaxation rather than fear with the problem object. Another aspect of the therapy teaches people to learn by positive reinforcement, or rewards, perhaps by getting something they enjoy as a reward for confronting the spider, or stopping smoking or binge-eating. While this method is particularly useful for children, many of us, especially those who are depressed, have taken all forms of self-reward from our lives.

Behaviour therapists may make a 'behavioural analysis', asking you to keep a record of what you want to change (for example, binge-eating or drinking alcohol or school refusal or depressed inactivity) in order to work out when it most often occurs, and perhaps to get some idea of what prompts it and what its consequences are. So from this record you might discover you always dive for the bottle when you've had a phone call from a parent; or that you eat vast quantities whenever the children leave to go to school. The idea of this form of behaviour therapy is not to answer why the problem occurred in the first place, but to change your pattern of living to make it more difficult to occur in the present, and to substitute some other more pleasant or appropriate activity for the problem one. Behaviour therapy may also include the introduction or the re-learning of skills, such as managing children or making love, or assertion training, where you are taught to stand up for yourself without aggression or guilt.

Cognitive-behavioural therapy uses these techniques but emphasises that it is also the way people think – the way they interpret events or label things – that affects their emotions and their behaviour. So thoughts such as, 'I never get anything right', or 'Nobody will ever love me', are likely to affect both mood and behaviour, in that the person may not attempt any task (including therapy!), or seek love or caring from anyone (including a therapist!).

Similarly, *the cause* that people give to events can strongly affect their mood and their behaviour: if you receive a blow on the back of the head and think it was a robber with a cosh you will probably feel afraid and may run away; if you think it was a boy throwing a rock you will be angry and turn to confront him; if you think it was a branch blown from a tree, you may simply be a bit fed up and rub your sore head. So our thoughts clearly affect our mood, and subsequently our actions. Cognitive therapists teach patients to challenge thoughts such as 'He's doing that because he doesn't like me', and to recognise when they wrongly label physical symptoms (for example, that the effects of over-breathing are the beginnings of a heart attack). This therapy is particularly successful with depressed people and with those who suffer panic attacks.

In the United Kingdom anyone can call themselves a psychotherapist and set themselves up in practice. This undoubtedly poses a problem if private therapy is required, and it's always better to go to someone recommended either by your doctor, or by another professional health worker, or by someone who has actually used the service. The long lists of strange initials which appear after the names of some people who have set themselves up in practice are extremely confusing and may be provided by completing very unsatisfactory courses.

Within the National Health Service only qualified people will be employed and some of these will practise psychotherapy. **Psychiatrists** are doctors who go on to specialise in the treatment of mental disorders. Relatively few of them have formal psychotherapy training, although this is increasing with the introduction of specialist departments of psychotherapy in some cities. **Clinical psychologists** spend three years as undergraduates studying psychology, where they learn the theoretical basis for their skills, followed by two to three years clinical training, often with an emphasis on behaviour therapy. This is sometimes followed by psychotherapy training. Other professionals who may have specialised experience or qualifications are **psychiatric social workers** and **nurses**. **Psychoanalysts** come from a variety of backgrounds, though principally from medical, psychological or social work. Their training invariably includes their own personal analysis. Psychoanalysis is usually private but, depending on where you live, may be obtained on the NHS; for example, at the

Tavistock Clinic in North London, provided you meet certain criteria.

Within the field of psychotherapy research, there is little debate that all these methods are effective. However, there is growing awareness that it is not just the technique which causes the change, but that the quality of the therapist and the relationship between the therapist and client is also very important. It is therefore perfectly possible that one therapist will 'suit' you better than another and you may decide not to settle with the first one if you have strong doubts about how well you'll get on. However, if you find yourself chopping and changing rather a lot, or going to two at once, you probably need to realise that sticking with one therapist, even if he or she seems less than perfect (which we all are), may be an important part of the therapy.

Akin to psychological help comes another group of therapies which work by letting people express themselves in some way, such as **art therapy** or **dance therapy** or **drama** or **music therapy**. **Occupational therapy** may be used to re-establish skills of living which may have deteriorated due to illness or to a long stay in hospital, and to help people to gain their independence.

PHYSICAL TREATMENTS

Physical treatments, including drugs and electro-convulsive therapy (ECT), may only be authorised by medically qualified people. It is their expertise with these that forms the main distinguishing role of psychiatrists; their advice is very important in deciding which drugs to use, especially when more than one is being taken.

Drugs are the most commonly used medical treatment, and by far the most prescribed group is that known as the benzodiazepines or **minor tranquillisers**, such as Valium and Librium. These are used in cases of stress and anxiety, for phobic conditions and panic attacks. They may be prescribed for sleep problems, and for a host of illnesses which the general practitioner considers may have a psychosomatic basis; that is, that the physical symptoms may be at least partly caused by stress or worrying or general anxiety. They are addictive so their power decreases quite rapidly within a few weeks, necessitating larger doses to maintain the same effect. For this reason it is usually considered nowadays that they should only be taken when really necessary, and used only for a short period to provide relief while people deal with the problem that is creating the symptoms. The details of the various drugs and their side-effects are dealt with in Chapter 4 on anxiety.

The second important group of drugs is the neuroleptics or **major tranquillisers**, such as Largactil and Modecate. These are used primarily in schizophrenia to control the primary symptoms, but may also be used for mania and some, in much smaller doses, for severe anxiety. They are discussed in detail in Chapter 13 on schizophrenia.

Antidepressant drugs are used, as the name suggests, to treat depression. Those most commonly prescribed are the tricyclic group which takes 10–14 days to become effective. The other group, used less often, is the monoamine oxidase inhibitors which can be dangerous if taken alongside certain foods. Some medication may be both antidepressant and anti-anxiety. These drugs are discussed in more detail in Chapter 6 on depression. Lithium, discussed in Chapter 14, is used as a preventative drug for manic-depression, and occasionally just for mania or depression.

Electroconvulsive therapy, or ECT, was first used when a doctor noticed that people with epilepsy did not seem to suffer from schizophrenia (in fact this was untrue), and so the aim was to produce a convulsive reaction in order to cure schizophrenia. Although this logic was both false and simplistic and failed, ECT was found to have a positive effect on some people suffering from severe depression, and that's its principal use today. More rarely it will be given to people with schizophrenia or mania, but its usefulness in these conditions is not generally accepted. Between 4 and 12 sessions (rarely more) of ECT are given, usually to in-patients. It involves passing an electric current through the brain from temple to temple under general anaesthetic and a muscle relaxant. Again, this is discussed in more detail in Chapter 6.

Finally, **psychosurgery** or leucotomy or lobotomy or functional neurosurgery are all names for surgery performed on the brain in order to relieve severe forms of obsessional disorders, depression or, extremely rarely, anxiety. It is understandably used very infrequently and certainly should not be contemplated unless all other forms of treatment, both physical and psychological, have been tried for a number of years, and by a number of people. Like ECT, there is very little idea how it works, or whether it is successful in the long term, and there is considerable debate about whether it should be performed at all.

HOSPITALISATION

Most people's fears concerning breakdowns come from images they have of psychiatric hospitals, or asylums, or 'funny farms' or 'looney bins'. On the whole these images have their basis in the Victorian establishments set in acres of grounds on the outskirts of most large cities. Deliberately built as a world apart, it was all too easy for fear of the unknown to grow in non-patients. Until the fifties, some of these fears had more than a vestige of reality to them, since wards were kept locked and treatments were often both primitive and experimental.

After World War II, various social and economic changes resulted in wards being unlocked and mental hospitals becoming very different places. Since then hospital stays have become shorter and shorter: over half leave in under a month, and over 90 per cent leave within a year. Nursing staff are no longer custodial, but well trained, and general hospitals now have psychiatric wards for short-stay patients. The plan in most parts of Britain is gradually to empty the old establishments and to treat people more and more within the community, in day centres or in their homes. This comes from the realisation that long stays in hospitals are not necessarily the best way to equip people for a more normal life outside, and so in-patient treatment is now kept to a minimum. However, it is important that local authorities and politicians are constantly reminded by patients, relatives and helpers that community care is expensive: it should continue to be regarded as the *better* option, *not* the cheaper one.

Most people enter hospital as voluntary patients, but about 5 per cent are detained compulsorily, or 'sectioned' under the Mental Health Act 1983.* The Act refers to 'mental illness' and allows for compulsory admission only where it's warranted, in the inter-

---

* This only applies in England and Wales. Slightly different regulations operate in Scotland and Northern Ireland.

est of the patient's own health or safety (for example, where someone is clearly threatening or attempting suicide, or where they're behaving in such a way as to provoke the aggression of others), or to protect others. There are many safeguards now to unnecessary detention, and orders for admission longer than 72 hours need two doctors, only one of whom is employed by the hospital. In emergencies one doctor only is necessary for admissions up to 72 hours, preferably one who knows the patient, and application is made by an approved social worker or nearest relative. There are many detailed provisions for rights in such cases, and patients and relatives can get information from social services or from their local MIND office.

Although a stay in hospital is not an end in itself, it may be necessary to give people a break from the environment that is engulfing them, and to teach them new skills of changing it or of coping within it. Most hospitals are able to provide more specialist services such as occupational therapy and art therapy, though these too are gradually moving towards a community-based service. The word 'asylum' means sanctuary or refuge, and this aspect of care will continue to have an important role to play in assisting peace of mind.

These treatments are not exclusive, but will often be used in various combinations. For example, someone admitted to hospital for severe depression may be given ECT to relieve the worst of the symptoms and then be put on a course of antidepressant medication, during which they may begin psychotherapy in order to explore what's happened to them and how things might be altered in the future.

Either within the hospital setting, or separately run by organisations such as the Richmond Fellowship, it is sometimes possible to be offered a place in a therapeutic community. This is a setting in which a group of patients and staff work together to provide sanctuary, to help each other towards an understanding of their problems, and to learn ways of changing. Wigoder's book *Images of Destruction* provides an account of his experiences in such a community.

Part Two

Chapter

3

Daily stress
and life events

Humans have always been subject to stress of some sort or another right back to the times when we huddled around our campfires in bearskins. The stress of daily living produced challenges which as a species we met and so extended our environments, our sophistication and our capabilities. That challenges are necessary to us is suggested by cultures where the environment has produced an easy living: their peoples still create their own demands by way of art or music or forms of competition. Both extremes of stress, whether too much (which we'll call pressure), or too little (which we'll call boredom) can spur us into activity to relieve or to increase the demands upon us. This is demonstrated by the figures on page 24. The first figure shows the Chinese symbols which represent the word 'stress'; the top symbol meaning 'danger' and the lower 'opportunity'.

The second figure, devised by Roy Payne, shows that stress has two negative ends, and we spend our time engineering our most satisfying existence somewhere around the middle.

However, we are all very different in how much outside pressure and demands, or how little boredom, we desire and can tolerate. This results partly from physical variations and partly from our life histories. What we call personality can be seen as a combination of the two. There is increasing evidence that people vary physiologically as a reaction to outside events and that some people, for whatever reason, more easily perceive threat in their environments

危
機

STRESS =

danger

opportunity

Fig. 1

than others. This may be something you are physically born with, or it may be the result of a long history of threat (physical or psychological) in the environment in which you grew up. For example, someone who has had a very critical parent who seemed impossible to please may carry with them right through adulthood both the need to please and a strong doubt about their capabilities. This will make having a boss who gives little feedback much more stressful than it would for someone who had been brought up to believe that they could do well, that they weren't always to blame

S	Submitted
T	Torpid
R	Relaxed
E	Energised
S	Stretched
S	Smashed

Fig. 2

when things went wrong, and that they could expect fair feedback if they asked for it.

Stress that is experienced negatively comes from actually having too few skills or resources to meet outside demands, or from thinking that you have too few. It may, of course, also come from having, or thinking that you have, too many, as in the case of many unemployed people who suffer frustration and boredom because of unused capabilities. There is abundant evidence now (much of which comes from Professor Peter Warr's team at Sheffield University) that people develop many of the physical and psychological problems of stress and even of breakdown when they lose their jobs. Young people assessed before they left school and again at regular intervals show that their symptoms of distress rise and fall, not in relation to how they were at school, but whether they have jobs or not. Many older people, especially men, tend to lose self-esteem when they lose their employment, but in younger people it's more a reaction to the sheer inactivity of being jobless. It is only when people can discover new challenges that their lives improve, as this quote from an article by Dr David Fryer of the University of Stirling shows. It's by someone who turned unemployment into something positive:

> *To me it's an opportunity, to be unemployed . . . I've used my unemployment as a sort of finding out time . . . I've discovered things in myself, gifts and abilities, that I never knew were there, that wouldn't have been discovered, definitely, not while I was (employed) because all I did (then) was sort of exist to get ready for the next day to exist through the next day.*
> (Unemployed teacher)

It is not the intermittent experience of pressure or boredom that causes problems, but an experience that is chronic or unending: a job where demand follows demand, providing neither rest nor satisfaction; a marriage where the wife is beaten for trying to make herself look appealing, and beaten when she doesn't; a home where parents never talk but will not separate for the children's sake; a job where every target that is achieved is then extended; a life where everyday survival brings an unemployed person constantly up against the barriers of officialdom.

And we can create our own chronic stresses too, as John, a retired manager, explained to me:

25

I'd fought my way up to the top of the firm, and when I got there I really felt flat. I went around creating new accounts, hardly ever delegating, really doing two jobs at once, but it still wasn't enough. So I started playing squash – not just the odd game, but with the same kind of determination that I faced work with. I hated losing and so filled up all my leisure time with improving my skills. And I had a heart attack. Hardly surprising, looking back.

When we experience a level of stress which is fairly continual and excessive, our bodies and our minds will usually produce clear warning signals, whether physical or psychological. Most of us suffer some of these symptoms of stress from time to time: it makes good sense that our bodies are designed to do this. In evolutionary terms it is only a short time ago that we needed to be able to gather together all our physical resources at a moment's notice in order to fight our prey or flee from our enemies; for example, we needed adrenalin to be released into our bodies in order to make our hearts pump harder and provide more oxygen for our limbs. For this we were given a second nervous system, one which is separate from that which controls our voluntary movements. For most of us, this so-called parasympathetic system is not under our conscious control but simply reacts to things which cause us fear. There are some indications however that yogis can control aspects of their systems, and research has shown that if you are given feedback (e.g. of your blood pressure) you can learn to alter activity in that part of the system.

Because evolutionary change takes so many millions of years, the reactions of our nervous systems have not caught up with the enormous changes in our lifestyles. Most of us no longer fight bears but many of us fear that we have failed in our ambitions, whether for fame, for fortune or for beauty. While we no longer flee from stronger tribes, we long sometimes to escape from the boss's frown. At times when our bodies are telling us we should vent our rage, social pressure tells us to smile politely and be grateful. Helpless in our armchairs we watch and feel fearful for ourselves and our families as we are bombarded with news of unemployment, of pollution, of hijackings and of nuclear annihilation. We fear different things, but we still fear, and our bodies still react in the same way as they did ten thousand years ago.

In the twentieth century the effects of all this are the physical and psychological symptoms of stress. These are set out in Figure 3 below:

Physical symptoms	Behavioural symptoms	Emotional symptoms
nausea	irritability	depression
cold sweats	increased alcohol	loss of confidence
dizziness	increased	worry
diarrhoea	cigarettes	irritability
backache	decreased sexual	preoccupation
appetite loss	desire	with physical
digestive	poor work	symptoms
problems	performance	restlessness
headaches	absenteeism	
chest pain	school refusal	
shaking	avoiding	
tingling	situations	
hair loss	avoiding social	
butterflies	contact	
dry mouth	concentration	
difficulty getting	loss	
breath	difficulty getting	
lightheadedness	to sleep	

Fig. 3

As you can see from the long list of common physical symptoms, most of these may exist without any psychological cause and so should always be checked up on by your doctor. It is also perfectly normal to experience any of them in a mild form or intermittently simply as a response to everyday pressure or boredom. Most of the time they are short-lived and tolerable; for example, as we try to park the car in a crowded street we feel our heart thumping more than usual; or as we have blood taken at the hospital we find ourselves feeling somewhat faint; or knowing it's our turn next to answer a question in the classroom we have a sudden pain shoot through our heads. Sometimes when our bodies provide too much adrenalin we engage in some other activity to use up some of the excess. Thus you will often see drivers scratching or touching their heads just after a manoeuvre involving danger. These are our individual responses to the stresses and strains of everyday life.

If one of these symptoms – for example, chest pain, headaches or impotence – occurs uncomfortably often people will usually contact their doctors thinking they have some illness such as an indeterminate virus, or heart disease, or a brain tumour. This is an essential first step whenever a physical symptom persists, but often it is only after exhaustive medical tests that people will accept that their conditions are to do with stress and that they need to change their lives in some way to reduce the stress.

On their own then, these symptoms are simply warning you that your body is under too much pressure. It is only when they appear irrespective of demands; when they continue so that everything you do begins to be affected, and when they start changing your behaviour so that perhaps you begin to avoid situations or people; it is only at this point, when things are beginning to feel beyond your control, that you can suspect a breakdown.

But, as John's story has shown, a nervous breakdown is only one aspect of extreme stress (just as extreme stress is only one thing that might be involved in a breakdown). It is probably true that we all have a weak point: it may be our hearts, or our stomachs, our colons, or our minds. Each one may be taxed to a point where we suffer coronary heart disease, or gastric ulcers, or spastic colons, or nervous breakdowns. In this way stress is seen as related to many illnesses, from eczema to cancer, from migraine to diabetes, from flu to schizophrenia, from asthma to depression.

There are many books on ways to relieve your stress. Some are general, some concentrate on stress at work, others on the stress of unemployment, and so on. But all of them propose three general ways that stress can be reduced:

1 You may alter the environment or your skills in dealing with it so that the level of demands is changed. So you might learn ways to feed both twins at once; or you might buy a computer to reduce the paperwork in a one-person business; or you may approach a women's refuge to gain support and escape

a battering husband. If your demands are too few, you may join a competitive club, or decide to begin an allotment or renovate a dilapidated house, or become involved politically, or learn how to knit so you can begin your own business.

2 You may alter the ways you think about and see the environment so it no longer seems so threatening whether the threat is from too much or too little pressure. One of Dr Fryer's subjects changed the way he viewed his lost job which in turn affected the way he saw his present unemployment:

At work you don't eat when you're hungry, you eat between one and two, 'cause that's when your dinner time is . . ., you go to bed at a certain time otherwise you're going to be very tired the next morning . . . for the last 30 years I've functioned within a framework that's been laid down by someone else.

(Unemployed steel worker)

Alternatively, you may change the way you see yourself so you no longer seem so incapable. Thus you may ask your boss if he or she is satisfied with your performance rather than always presuming a frown to be displeasure. It's surprising how many people then find that what they took to be a critical look was actually a headache, or resulted from the fact that the boss was also feeling under pressure. Even if you get negative feedback, it's never as bad as what's been going on in your head. Or you may change your views and see that unemployment is politically caused, rather than personally, and so your self-esteem should not be lowered; that your feelings of failure are caused by an economic system which requires you to never feel satisfied with yourself, rather than by your own inferiority.

3 You may teach yourself ways to cope with an unchangeable environment – having tested carefully which bits can be changed and which can't. This can be done by improving your general health with diet, exercise and deciding not to smoke and to reduce your alcohol intake; by learning how to relax and to put pleasure into your life in whatever way you

can. Some of the possible strategies are described in the self-help section in Chapter 4 on anxiety.

LIFE EVENTS

I've used the word 'stress' to refer to the daily pressures which at their best help us to gain satisfaction, meet challenges, learn and grow, and at their worst can help to cause both physical and psychological breakdown. 'Life events' is the term given to single stressors – to the changes in our lives, usually negative but sometimes positive, some of which are major and very disrupting, and some minor and overlapping with the daily hassles we call stress. An interest in the relationship between life events and illness began in the sixties, and since then quite sophisticated measurements have taken place to allow us to predict which events will have the most impact on the individual. However, just as with stress, which individuals will respond most to life changes, and which way they will respond is by no means clear.

Again, as with chronic stress, life events have been linked to a wide variety of disorders, both physical and psychological – not just to catching the odd virus, but also to cancer, heart disease and depression. When someone said, 'She died of a broken heart', they may have been very close to reality. Each type of life event is, in research, given a weighting, and the sum of these weightings over a period of time shows how likely it is that you will suffer some unspecified illness. For example, if you get divorced and leave your home, and people in your family get ill, and it's Christmas . . . this will almost double your chances of illness in the next six months.

The most significant life events are those which involve some loss; so death of a spouse heads the list, followed by divorce or separation, death of others who are close, then losing one's job, serious illness, and so on. Even events which are generally thought to be pleasant, such as marriage, or the birth of a child, or moving to a better job or home, all involve a cost on the life events score sheet, perhaps because even these involve a loss in some way – a loss of freedom, or of former colleagues and friends.

Many of these life changes are to a large extent unavoidable, but wherever possible it is advisable not to bring too many of them together at one time since that will raise your score unnecessarily. So don't move house or change jobs just as you have your first baby, or very soon after the loss of someone close.

Major life events have stronger links to experiencing a nervous breakdown than any of the daily pressures or boredom earlier described. This is partly because some events are thought, in the right circumstances, to actually precipitate a breakdown, though there is generally some other factor involved as well; for example, Brown and Harris' research on working-class women has shown that many of those suffering a major loss have become depressed, but only if they have no one in whom to confide. Other factors which intervened in this way to make the woman vulnerable to major events included having a number of pre-school children, having no job, or losing their mother before the age of eleven. Similarly research suggests that some people and not others will develop psychological problems after a major event because they have a particular way of thinking about things; for example, that they see the happenings in their lives as primarily caused by themselves in some way, rather than as a result of outside circumstances or other people.

There is no doubt that, when major events occur, people often go pell-mell through the whole gamut of psychological disorders, but usually their reactions are short-lived. For example, Pat's husband announced one night over coffee that he had been having an affair for the past year and he intended to leave Pat for the woman involved. He then proceeded to pack his bags and, within an hour, had left. Pat watched him stunned:

I remember feeling little bursts of controlled anger, but that's all. I made a few sneering remarks about how she might not tolerate his smelly feet or his snoring, but on the whole I felt almost nothing. Well nothing in comparison to what followed. The next day my young son knocked over a vase of flowers and I screamed at him and then began to cry and cry. Eventually I pulled myself together and went back to feeling angry. Then I began to think of them both, eating their meals together, in bed together, having fun. He'd told me she was fun and I wasn't any more. The thoughts went on and on, day and night. I even planned their murder!

From then on Pat began to go through one phase after another.

At first, as if in a full-blown obsessional disorder, she couldn't stop herself thinking about them in very disturbing ways, and about what she could do to harm them. She talked of nothing else to her friends who at first were very supportive and angry themselves, but who later became a little alarmed at the extent of her rage and her threats. She suffered from a host of anxiety symptoms – lost her appetite, couldn't sleep, was shaking and had no concentration for anything but her thoughts. She found that if her anger stopped for a moment, as when she acknowledged to herself that she still loved him, she was flooded with depression and simply wanted to die. She found herself with violent thoughts of suicide that both comforted her and terrified her.

> *At the time I wondered (though I didn't much care) if I was going mad. I think my friends wondered this too! It all lasted at its most ferocious for about a month, and then suddenly there were days when things seemed different. My mood would change to something other than anger or despair; I'd find myself appreciating some flowers, or the sunshine, or laughing at something the kids said. Over a period of about three months, the moods gradually went. I now can appreciate how good life can be without him. I guess I take a little delight as I see him behaving in just the same aggressive ways with her as he did with me, but I'm certainly not thinking all the time about dreadful things that might happen to either of them. I feel lonely sometimes and sad about losing the good times we used to have, but I guess we lost those a long time before he actually left.*

GRIEF

When you lose someone you care about, you go through a period of grieving during which time you may well feel the pain will never end. As Pat's experience showed, the pain has all the hallmarks of a nervous breakdown: anxiety, depression, obsessionality, a touch of anorexia, and perhaps some paranoia. People whose loved ones have died will sometimes see them or feel them in the room, and this will add to their worries, or the worries of their friends and relatives that they are going out of control. The important difference is that in the vast majority of cases this will eventually end without help from outside sources, though other people can speed the process along by letting the person talk about their loss. Occasionally people do get stuck in the mourning process, and then professional help may be needed.

It is generally accepted that there are four tasks or stages to grieving. How long it will take an individual to work his or her way through the tasks will vary enormously according to the person concerned, the relationship that's ended, and the support and friendship that surrounds the one who's grieving. It may be one year; it may be two, and perhaps considerably more to feel competent and stable once again.

The first task is to accept the fact that the loss has taken place. This can be clearer in death than in marital separation, and funerals certainly help to force the reality upon people. Denying death can be perfectly normal for a short period, but continuing to do it (for example, by keeping a child's room for years just as it was before he or she died) can make a person stuck even in the first stage. Another way around this is to pretend to yourself that you never cared much anyway, so a friend of mine simply left her dead husband in hospital, saying: 'You deal with him. He'd have hated any fuss.'

Second, you have to really let yourself experience the pain which is both physical and emotional. People are sometimes slowed down in this stage by well-meaning friends who feel they should try to stop the tears rather than let them flow. It can be quickly communicated to the person concerned that tears and anguish make others uncomfortable and should be repressed. Although they may be necessary in the first few days, tran- quillisers will have the same effect as saying 'There, don't cry', and simply slow down the grieving process.

Part of the painful feelings you experience may contain anger, and, while this may be easily given vent to in separation or divorce, it is sometimes difficult to express angry, hurt feelings about someone who has died. At some stage these need to be acknowledged so that the full loving memory, warts and all, can be allowed to exist.

The third task is to adjust to living without the person. People provide a number of roles for each other, both practical and emotional, and this stage requires the learning of new knowledge and skills. Norma had not worked since her husband took early retirement. Whereas he would walk each evening to spend an hour with friends at the local, she was content to depend solely on him for her company. He organised all the financial aspects and did most of the practical tasks around the house. Those he couldn't do, he knew the best people to ask. His death left Norma feeling totally hopeless.

> *My first reaction on dealing with anyone like tradespeople, or the pension office, or the bank, or even neighbours who were trying to be friendly, was to believe they were trying to rob me. No one could be trusted. In fact, there were elements of truth in this, and that's probably what made me so paranoic. People kept coming to the house asking if I would be selling; and a couple from the village asked if I still wanted my car – all that sort of thing. The feeling became so bad that I wouldn't let my son help me with my finances because I thought he would steal my money if I let him see what I'd got. Dreadful, looking back.*
>
> *But in some ways all this made me learn to become independent much faster, and by the time I'd learnt to trust people again, I'd also learnt a lot of new skills! At first it would make me sad to do things myself, because I would remember Jack doing them. But then gradually I began to enjoy the confidence I got by knowing what was what. There's so much that we leave our partners to do, and it really is a mistake. It makes life so much more frightening when they've gone.*

The final task is to leave emotionally the one you've lost, so that you are able to begin another relationship if the right person comes along. People become stuck at this stage for a number of reasons; for example, they don't want to risk being hurt again by starting with someone new; or they feel disloyal to their dead partner by beginning again. Although remarriage after divorce is quite high, after bereavement it's really very low, and this is likely to be because people refuse to complete this final task. Remarriage is, of course, no indication of health, but it is possible to get stuck with lost relationships other than marriage: sometimes adolescents may find it difficult to start having friends of the opposite sex after they have lost a parent of that sex. 'For about five years', one young man told me, 'I wouldn't have a girlfriend for more than one or two dates. It felt as if I was betraying Mum in some way. It took a lot of persistence on Jane's part to get me out of that!' They clearly won't be experiencing a nervous breakdown just by refusing to contemplate other relationships; they are simply denying themselves further possibilities of love.

Because life stress, whether continuous hassles or major single events, can make you vulnerable to a variety of disorders, both physical and psychological, there is no clear boundary between these situations and those that follow. The moment when a person decides that things have become out of control will very much depend on them, and also upon those close to them, upon their doctor, and the facilities for help in the area in which they live. It will also depend upon their knowledge, and the aim of the following chapters is to provide you with sufficient knowledge so that you will know when things are going wrong – at which points chronic stress or the aftermath of life events can be seen as anxiety disorders or depression, when safeguards against fear become obsessional–compulsive disorders, when drinking alcohol to relieve the symptoms of stress turns into an addiction. It will help you to judge when to go for help and what help may be offered.

Chapter

Anxiety states and panic

Stephen had been an electrician in the coal industry since he was in his teens. Now in his mid-thirties, he had recently been promoted to a managerial position on the surface and had overall responsibility for electrical work for the whole pit. He was on call 24 hours a day and he found himself worrying constantly about what was happening when he was away from the pit. He felt very tense all the time and whenever the phone went his heart crashed inside him and he felt sick. He'd cut down his social life quite considerably. One morning before breakfast he was called to the site to oversee a problem with the lighting in a new shaft:

> *It was a fairly routine problem; no one's fault in particular, though looking back I think I always had twinges of guilt whenever anything went wrong. Anyway, it wasn't hard for me to fix it. But walking from the mine to the pit manager's office, I felt the earth spin suddenly. My legs were wobbling away like jelly and I was sure I was going to faint. I managed to get to the car and lay down on the back seat with the doors locked, praying no one would see me. I was shaking like a leaf all over.*

Gradually the frightening sensations subsided and he decided to drive home and spend the day in bed: it must be a virus of some kind, he thought. The next morning he felt fine, but as he had his breakfast and got ready for work he could feel himself becoming very tense and apprehensive. As he began driving, the same symptoms happened again and he pulled over to the side of the road. When he felt better he drove to his doctor who told him to stay off work for the rest of the week. 'Is it a virus?' Stephen asked. 'Could be,' answered his doctor.

During the following week he was aware of the knot in his stomach and the vague feeling something dreadful might happen. But on the whole he felt quite a lot better until his boss rang to ask how he was. Again his stomach churned and he felt sick. The night before he was due to return to work he couldn't sleep at all and in the morning went straight to the doctor's once again. 'Is anything worrying you in your job?' she asked. 'No more than usual,' he replied. When, after a few weeks, his wife realised that he was fearing even to go into the garden, she and the doctor managed to convince him he needed psychological help.

It's likely that Stephen had been suffering from a mild anxiety state for some time before he had the panic attack that made him and others notice something wrong. He had been suffering many of the physical symptoms of stress and had experienced feelings of foreboding which had made him begin to change his social life a little.

Any of the symptoms of stress described on p. 27 can be present during anxiety. During his panic attack, Stephen experienced a large number of the physical symptoms all at once. This can be so terrifying that people need to leave wherever they are at the time – a meeting, a theatre, the supermarket – and are often convinced that they are going to die, or at least to faint. Not everyone's anxiety state begins so dramatically. For some people the symptoms simply get stronger over time; or else they presume they would get more severe if they did not avoid the situations that seem to make things worse.

It is not the panic attack alone, nor the more generalised symptoms that make people wonder if this is a nervous breakdown; it's the fact that they change as a result of the experience. Filled with a sense of apprehension without apparent cause, they change their behaviour in some way, as Stephen did, perhaps by beginning to avoid the situation that appeared to precipitate the attack. In his case he put it down to the pressures of the job. Whatever actually caused those first symptoms, they are perpetuated by a fear of their repetition.

It is when the sense of apprehension or the fear of these physical sensations is so severe or so continuous that it starts to change your life in some inappropriate way (for example, by avoiding certain situations) that you know you are suffering from an anxiety state.

Others around you may well be noticing things are going wrong, but they have only the behavioural symptoms to go by. The list in Figure 3 (p. 27) is by no means exhaustive, but basically what we notice is some change for the worse in a person's behaviour: they become *more* irritable and withdrawn, they work *less* well, they seem to be avoiding certain situations, especially social ones. A common way to avoid things that cause fear is by taking drugs – prescribed drugs such as tranquillisers; forbidden drugs such as marihuana; or, most commonly of all, alcohol.

Sometimes the change that occurs is dramatically swift, but often it is gradual and more difficult to recognise. If someone close to you is being particularly hard to get on with, it takes some effort to remember that they weren't like that a couple of months ago, let alone a couple of years. Because we are involved in the relationship we will often see the change in terms of ourselves, and explain it in terms of rejection and hurt. When a person is physically ill it is easy to respond to them still, however damaged their bodies might be, because their minds are behaving in the same way. But when someone is hurting emotionally it often appears that they have changed in some fundamental manner, and it's all too easy to feel hurt by them and to resent them for becoming so different.

Like the changes in behaviour, the emotional symptoms of anxiety are again secondary to the physical ones. If your life is beginning to feel out of control because you can no longer do some important part of it because of your feelings of dread or in case your symptoms reappear, you are, not surprisingly, going to lose confidence in yourself, and perhaps become irritable with others as you deal with your worry and tension. You are likely to become very preoccupied with what's happening in your body and will often lose concentration as you try to attend to what your heart is doing or whether the tingling has returned to your fingers. Others may feel so helpless about the anxiety that seems to come from nowhere, and so hopeless that anything will cure it that they will become depressed. Depression and anxiety very often are seen together but when this happens it is often the anxiety which arrived first.

To come back to Stephen, he experienced a full panic attack

early on in his anxiety state. Whether it starts so dramatically or whether the symptoms just seem to get gradually worse over time, the important thing is that people begin to change their behaviour in some way in order to avoid the fear.

Stephen saw his symptoms in physical terms. He explained them away to himself and others as simply being a virus. Although they reappeared with any contact with work, he still denied that things had not been too good for some time and tried to bluff himself that he was just not well. At first he found that a night at the pub made him forget things altogether; feeling even worse the next day was worth it for those few hours free of worrying and trembling and also he was often able to put things down to the hangover itself. But gradually even walking to the gate produced some dizziness and he became afraid that he might faint one night in front of the lads. From then on he sat at home. Over this period of a couple of months his wife watched him becoming withdrawn and depressed. She heard him making excuses on the phone for why they wouldn't be able to go to this and that. She realised that although he was very often irritable with her, he didn't really want her to leave him alone. He wasn't her man any more, and she went to the doctor to ask for help.

It's important to understand that it's not the physical symptoms alone that create the anxiety state, but rather how you interpret the symptoms and what you do, or don't do, as a result of that interpretation. For example, there are two somewhat rarer sensations which are occasionally part of someone's anxiety state: depersonalisation and derealisation. In the latter you feel as if things around you are unreal, almost like a stage set, as if you're detached from the world in some way. Many people recognise this as a symptom of severe tiredness, make sure they get some rest, and think no more about it. For others it may fit the way they are thinking about themselves and then it can become something to be terrified about and anxiety can set in.

For example, Jock recently returned to Britain after five years in Kenya. He'd made the decision rather on the spur of the moment, and felt less than certain that it was a good move as each day he faced the grey cold of an English January:

I didn't let myself say, Jock, you've made a wee mistake, but you can go

39

back if you want. That might have been helpful. Instead, I'd go out boozing each night with anyone I could find. I let myself get very tired and low, and started getting this sense each morning that I was living in some cardboard cut-out of a world: not even in colour, just black and white and grey. It became very scary because it made me feel trapped in unreality, which actually I must have been feeling anyway, but not letting myself acknowledge it.

In depersonalisation people begin to feel *they* are unreal, that their bodies are not a part of them, that they are on the outside looking in, or something like that. Once again, it can be transitory and put down to tiredness, or it can be seen as terrifying.

Leslie was a policewoman on the drug squad and had been married about a year when she began an affair with a fellow officer. It was very much a sexual attraction, rather than love. Her husband still did not know, and she was feeling guilty and constantly worried. After a week on night-shift she experienced the feeling that her mind and body were separate, that she didn't own her body. She found this terrifying and the more frightened she felt the worse it seemed to become and the more she began to suffer other signs of anxiety. Perhaps it would have been helpful if someone had pointed out to her at the time that not owning her body might be something she almost wanted, since the actions of her body had been disturbing her life and making her so guilty, and that is why the sensation had so much meaning for her.

Many people who suffer from panic and anxiety over-breathe or hyperventilate; that is, they breathe too fast which leads to too little carbon dioxide in the blood. This produces all the physical symptoms that are linked to anxiety: believe me, if you pant hard now you'll quickly know what I mean. But once again, these are simply the physical reactions to over-breathing; they are only the symptoms of anxiety when you become afraid of them. If you ask someone to hyperventilate deliberately, knowing what's causing their symptoms, they usually do not find them particularly unpleasant. In someone who doesn't know why it's occurring, those same sensations can feel like you're dying which will produce blind terror, which in turn can lead to more hyperventilation and so on (see p. 47).

WHY DID IT HAPPEN?

When people seek help for anxiety, one of the first things many of them ask is, 'Why me?'. If they are in a stressful work situation, they may be able to point to aspects of the job which might be thought to put an intolerable load on anyone, but they can equally well point to others suffering the same load who have survived the strain. If they are unemployed they see themselves as having no particular pressures, apart from the financial ones shared by millions. In fact, they agree, they'd really welcome a bit of pressure. If they are rich, employed, with a spouse, family and everything that society told them they should achieve to be really happy, then they often feel particularly guilty. It seems totally unreasonable that, even in the lap of luxury, they should be anxious and unhappy.

We all look for explanations of the illnesses that happen to us: if we have a cold we'll often decide when and where we caught it: 'It was that man I sat next to on the bus last Friday, coughing and sneezing everywhere,' or, 'I should have worn a scarf when I walked down to the shops.' Even people suffering from cancer will try to find a reason: 'I had a lot of X-rays when I broke my leg as a child,' or, 'My mother and my uncle both died of cancer,' or, 'Johnny thumped me there when I was little.' While we have a great many explanations, both from folklore and from science, about the causes of physical illnesses, we have far fewer to explain the mysteries of mental problems.

But we still have a need to find a cause. With anxiety, as your life appears more and more difficult to control, knowing the reasons for your symptoms may allow you to place some order on what feels like chaos. Explanations, such as the effects of over-breathing described above, can therefore provide considerable relief. However, we sometimes choose an explanation that masks the problem or stops us dealing with it rather than exposing it. Sarah's story illustrates this:

> *I was standing in the pub next to Matt. It was crowded and the music was loud. I guess I was still tired from staying up too late the night before, but I always enjoyed this band. Matt had a friend with him from his university days, and I'd been vaguely thinking what a lot of friends he had, and how I didn't know most of them. Not surprising*

really; we'd had what they call a whirlwind romance and had only been married three weeks. I'd been on a working holiday from Canada – just doing any odd job that came along really because I couldn't use my legal training in this country. Matt hadn't fancied Canada, and we were in love, so I'd decided to stay here with him. Matt looked down at me and smiled and whispered he loved me. I remember smiling back sort of automatically, and then the thought going through my mind, 'Well, I don't love you!' The next second my stomach turned over, my heart seemed to crash inside, and the room spun round. I thought I was dying. I came out in a cold sweat and had to rush to the lavatory. It was the most terrifying thing that had ever happened to me. And yet in some peculiar way I felt ashamed and quite clear that I had to keep it a secret.

Over the next few months she stayed in an almost perpetual state of anxiety, shaking inside and out, hardly eating or sleeping. To give meaning to her symptoms, she began to think God was punishing her, probably for divorcing her first husband and marrying Matt. She'd never been religious and knew this was crazy, but everything seemed crazy at the time. That God was punishing her seemed the most rational explanation; if it wasn't true then she was pretty sure she was going mad.

Sarah, newly married to a man she loved dearly and for whom she had chosen to give up her career and her home and parents still in Canada, couldn't let herself choose a cause that was linked directly to her marriage. Hadn't the symptoms actually started the moment she had a cross thought about her husband? No wonder she did not dare to touch this area again! Although somewhat bizarre, it was safer to use God and punishment as an explanation. Unfortunately, while she clung to this, there was little that could be done to help her and nothing she could do to help herself. In her case she needed an outsider to point out alternative reasons, and to help her to see that she could feel anger and still love Matt.

Stephen put his symptoms down to the stress of the job, and there was no doubt that the amount of responsibility he shouldered and the number of hours he was on call, were truly formidable. But while he saw it as only the job and not involving also his reaction to it, it was impossible to change anything. Although he persisted in his explanation, deep down he was beginning to admit to himself that not being able even to go for a drive into the country had little to do with the work situation.

In fact, although we all want explanations for our symptoms, we don't always need them in order to get back to normal. Although it often provides some relief to be given a cause that makes sense, it's rarely enough in itself. Knowing the probable reason for so much distress will often make clearer what should be done to stop the symptoms happening again, but the explanations will vary according to the treatment that you choose.

Many people put mental disorders down to heredity or at least to something physical within the body. For example, you often hear people say: 'Her mother suffered with her nerves too. It seems to run in the family,' or, 'He always was a nervous little boy.' It may well be true that we do inherit dispositions or physical characteristics which might predispose us to feeling anxious, but there is still no actual scientific basis known for this. Though we can often see nervous behaviour in several members of a family, living with an anxious parent will not be easy for any child and they may well have become anxious themselves not from heredity but from the environment in which they were brought up. Moreover, both anxiety and depression occur in the most unlikely people as well as those we might predict would suffer – the most macho man who's run his own business for years, or the most capable woman who could always be relied upon to help others.

The major problem with any purely physical explanation of anxiety is that, apart from giving pills which over time will have less and less effect, it would appear that there is nothing you can do about it. You were born with it, so that's all! Not very encouraging and also completely against the evidence which shows that by far the majority of people can be helped.

Another more useful explanation is that something from earlier in your life made you more likely to suffer anxiety in certain circumstances. The simplest form of this would be a person with a phobia about dogs (see Chapter 5) who had loved them until she was bitten at the age of three. Unfortunately such straightforward connections are very rare. More often what occurred in early life was some way of relating within the home in which you grew up, which has left you more likely to see threats in your environment, or with statements or rules about yourself – now so much part of you that you can hardly recognise them – which if challenged or broken can cause anxiety.

43

These statements might be that you only deserve love if you are successful at something; or that it's your job to make people happy; or that if you make a mistake you deserve to be ridiculed. These rules might be that you should never show your anger or your tears, that you should be a 'real man' or a 'real woman', and generally that you should behave in a particular way. It's the 'should' and 'must' that give the clue to a life rule. Of course we needed rules when we were young, and all parents set them to a greater or lesser extent. But when it felt as if, should the rule be broken, all the love would go, then the way is paved to anxiety.

In Sarah's childhood no one became angry. They sulked or they stewed or they took themselves to their rooms; their parents might stop speaking to the children or to each other, but no one was angry. So when Sarah had that small grumpy thought about Matt it was really the strongest indication she had had about the strength of her anger at being presumed – never even asked – that she would give up so much for him. Just as it's very difficult to get the cork back into the bottle of champagne when a little of the gas has escaped, so Sarah's violent symptoms erupted when she let out just a puff of her rage. Very few of these pent-up feelings belonged to Matt; most of them would be the result of years of frustration as a child. Part of Sarah's recovery eventually involved finding appropriate ways to deal with anger in the future.

Although it is quite possible that simply breaking one of these old rules would be enough on its own to cause distress, depending on the strength of feeling that was once attached to it, it's more usual that other physical events coincide. Both Sarah's and Stephen's defences to anxiety were undoubtedly lowered by their being tired, and you'll notice you are more likely to suffer if you've not been eating properly or had enough sleep or been generally getting too much of the high life.

The work of Professor Andrew Matthews and his colleagues in London shows that anxious people are more aware of threatening things within the environment than are those who are not anxious. While it is possible that there is a physical or genetic explanation for this, it is not difficult to see how people growing up in a threatening environment (whether this is the high rise ghettoes of our inner cities, or the presence of a constantly critical parent in the leafy suburbs) may learn to perceive threats more easily than those more fortunate.

Very occasionally a forerunner of an anxiety state is a bad experience on drugs such as marihuana or LSD or 'magic' mushrooms. Such an experience might be physically similar to a panic attack and, despite never touching drugs again, might be followed by bouts of general anxiety, not usually connected by the sufferer to the original episode. This is rare, but worth remembering for those with even a brief period of misspent youth.

Other events which may make you more vulnerable to anxiety and also to depression are changes in your life (Chapter 3). While changes concerning loss, such as divorce or separation, or death or illness, or unemployment, are most closely linked to psychological problems, even positive events such as a new house or marriage or a baby can cause strain. It's amazing how many people who come for help belittle the extent of the events that have happened to them.

> 'All I did was break my wrist,' said Rob, a clerk in an employment bureau. 'And I found myself waking up each morning feeling sick, and couldn't eat and shaking all over.'
>
> 'Had anything else been happening around that time?' his psychologist asked.
>
> 'Not really,' he sat looking puzzled. 'Job was difficult of course, because we'd just changed offices. I'd been promoted you see, and I wasn't feeling too sure about things.' He paused again. 'And I'd moved house, and the finances were a bit tricky. But I'd done that before. Not on top of keeping up payments on another house as well though, I suppose.'
>
> 'Another house?'
>
> 'Well, yes. My wife's in the other place with the kids and her new feller. Happened a few months back.'

And so on. Certainly such a list of life events, however common each is individually, might make someone vulnerable to anxiety and to depression. With physical illness scientists are beginning to suggest that we may all of us carry the potential to contract a disease, even cancer, but that it needs particular life circumstances to bring it out. Some of these will be avoidable, like smoking or drinking excessively, or less avoidable, like having an overload of daily stresses and strains, or completely unavoidable, like losing a parent.

The same thing is probably true about psychological distress. None of us have had perfect upbringings and none of us will give them to our own children. We can only try to be good enough. Given that, it is quite likely that we also carry within most of us the potential to suffer anxiety or depression, but it's only when later events come together in a particular way that we actually break down.

But what might cause anxiety in the first place will be only part of what keeps it going. It would be perfectly possible to have one panic attack, for example, and never again to suffer another anxiety symptom. What happens after the initial symptoms are experienced is to quite a large extent a fear of fear.

Stephen felt fine when he reached home after his initial frightening experience walking across towards the pit office to see his boss. Humans learn extremely fast and Stephen's mind and body between them decided that the work situation (or the boss, or possibly open spaces) made him suffer the symptoms of fear; home on the other hand enabled him to feel safe and relatively relaxed. From then on anything connected with work increasingly made the symptoms reappear and this gradually spread wider and wider so that driving the car and eventually even leaving the house became equally frightening.

Clark and Salkovskis, psychologists in Oxford, have put forward a very useful model concerning the causes of panic and anxiety. They proposed that when something threatens us (and why we feel threatened doesn't matter in this model), our natural reaction of fear makes *some* of us over-breathe. This causes a decrease in carbon dioxide in the blood which in turn causes some of the physical feelings we associate with anxiety. If we realise this is simply the result of over-breathing we will not panic or become anxious, but without this knowledge it's easy to become increasingly afraid. Figure 4 illustrates this vicious cycle which can lead to panic.

This fear of fear is therefore one of the first things to tackle if you are to overcome a general state of anxiety. You need to learn that anxiety is controllable, and that it doesn't need to go on for ever.

A model of the development of a panic attack*

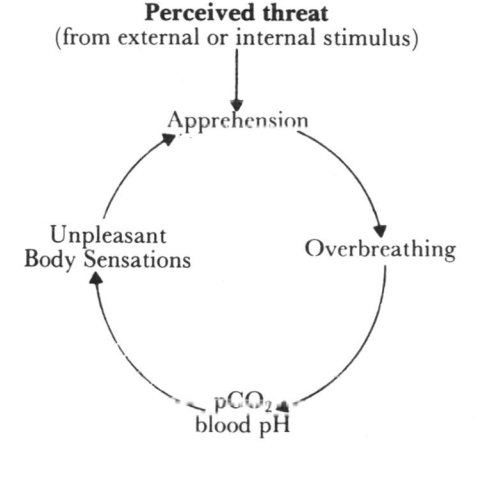

Fig. 4

WHAT CAN BE DONE?

Helping yourself

Research shows that a large proportion of people who develop anxiety find their symptoms fade with time, without any form of outside help. Although this is not a self-help book, this section describes ways that you can speed up this self-recovery.

If your anxiety symptoms are still fairly recent, or if you have learned to live with them without changing your life too much, then you may well be able to take measures yourself to end them or at least to make them considerably more bearable. Even if you decide that you need professional help, these strategies will be a useful adjunct to other forms of therapy.

It's always helpful as a start to buy yourself a small notebook and to use it as a record of the activities that eventually bring about recovery. Use the first page to write down things you did before you began suffering anxiety but that you no longer do or

* Clark, D.M., Salkovskis, P.M., Chalkley, A.J. (1985). *Journal of Behaviour Therapy and Experimental Psychiatry*, **16**, no 1, 23.

that you do more rarely. Decide which of these you wish you could put back into your life and use this list as one set of targets to achieve. At the back of the notebook write a list of the symptoms that distress you most, and use this for the target problems you most want to end. Give each problem a severity score of between 0 and 10, and your aim will be to reduce these initial scores to much smaller ones.

There is no one method to set about ending anxiety, and so you have to turn yourself into the scientist and find out what works best for you. But undoubtedly some things will be common to most sufferers, and these concern general health strategies. When you feel constantly anxious you will probably find yourself eating less, sleeping less, getting less exercise and, if you smoke, doing it more than ever. These are the first things to remedy. If you find yourself with no appetite, still make sure at least that you eat small tasty and nourishing meals – good soups, salads, fruits, milk, etc. Find out what slips down most easily for you and eat little and often. This is not the time for junk food.

Lack of sleep can feel an insurmountable problem and the worries and terrors that come in the night can make the anxiety seem even worse. Once again, there will be different strategies for different people: hot milk or sleep-inducing herb teas before you go to bed; a smaller or larger evening meal (try both and try different types of food); less television and more reading; a brisk walk shortly before bedtime. Try each strategy and note down any differences they produce, even very small ones. Don't expect huge changes and remember that one of the worst things about insomnia is lying there expecting a good eight hours and worrying about each one that passes. You'll probably feel better if you get up and have another hot drink, or read for a while. If worrying keeps you awake, write the worry down as it appears and promise yourself you'll consider it in the morning.

As we become more and more sedentary, scientists are increasingly appreciating the value of regular exercise both for our physical and our mental health and many people find it relieves both anxiety and depression. Decide to build some exercise into each day, and again try a variety to see which you most enjoy and which seems to make your symptoms reduce. Make sure you record both the successes and the failures since from the latter you are gaining vital information to enable things to improve. Try swimming, running, brisk walking and any sport that is available to you; join a keep-fit class or a yoga class and practise too at home. Research shows that exercise clearly has a beneficial influence on our nervous systems, lifting the mood, increasing relaxation and providing us with a sense of achievement which is important to raise sagging confidence.

Apart from these basic health strategies, by far the most common method used to control anxiety directly is relaxation. It is often possible to find classes for this (for example, from your local MIND Association), or to buy a special tape and teach it to yourself. There is an appendix at the end of this book which describes my own method of relaxation, part of which can be read into a tape-recorder to provide your own personal tape. It is important to remember that relaxation is not doing nothing; it's doing something very important. With it you are re-learning to use your tight tense muscles in a different way so they become relaxed whenever you need. Like all skills – typing, bricklaying, playing the piano – it requires regular and frequent practice, and you should aim at two sessions a day for the first few months.

Regular sessions of relaxation are useful in themselves but they will not cure anxiety on their own, in addition they must gradually be used as a means to let you confront what you fear, starting from situations that create the least anxiety and working towards those that cause the most. Using a friend to help you face your fears will make the experience less terrifying, though eventually you must do it alone. After each try, write down a score for your chosen achievements and for your symptoms. The most important thing you need to learn from these records is that fear is controllable, so that you can learn to reduce your fear of fear.

Margaret had been oppressed by a growing feeling of apprehension for several months. Often this was made more concrete by worrying about her house or her job or her family, but she was beginning to realise that, even when she could find nothing to worry about, she was feeling panicky. There seemed to be a continuous knot inside her and her heart would often miss a beat or pound for no apparent reason. She often felt dizzy while out shopping and she was sleeping poorly. Both at home and at the school where she taught she had noticed herself becoming unusually irritable. One day, in response to a child throwing a note across the room, she ran down the aisle, crashed her fist down on his desk, picked up all his books and threw them around the room, and then burst into tears. On the advice of her head teacher, she took herself straight to the doctor and asked for tranquillisers.

'I'm not sure that that would be really very useful', said her doctor. 'Why don't I give you a fortnight's sick leave instead, and use it to rest and see if things get better. Try and get yourself healthy. Things like that.'

His instructions sounded vague, but Margaret felt relieved that he'd regarded her as needing rest while at the same time he clearly felt she wasn't going mad – a thought that had crossed her mind rather often lately! Although she knew that things were beginning to get out of hand, she could also see clearly that she was letting them. She and Jim, her husband, didn't seem to talk much any more, and their sex life was almost non-existent. She spent her time either at school or hunched over in the armchair watching television, smoking, and worrying about her health. She suddenly felt quite optimistic that things could change.

The first thing I did was talk to my husband. Tell him what had been happening to me. He was wonderful. He was so relieved because he thought it was all to do with him in some way and he'd been feeling pretty miserable himself. Then we both decided what we'd like to change, just easy things like going out somewhere nice once a week, and getting the odd weekend away. We decided we'd both give up smoking and spend what we saved on things like that. And we did it. In the short-term I decided to get myself in trim and I joined a keep-fit class and a yoga class. The yoga was brilliant because it helped me to relax as well, and I've kept that up regularly.

I've tried all sorts of things to get me to sleep better, but eventually I found that a hot bath and warm milk and honey seemed to do the trick. I improved my diet a lot too and in fact I think this helped me feel fitter and made stopping smoking not so bad. Gradually the awful knot that had been inside me for so long started unravelling. Sometimes it seemed to tighten up again, but at least I knew what to do about it. If it was in the day I'd take myself out for a walk at lunchtime. If it was in the evening I'd take myself to bed with a hot water-bottle and a hot drink and a good book – or even with my husband! – and gradually this was enough to make it go. Even the worrying was much less; I think I needed worries just to explain to myself why I felt so anxious all the time. It probably took about three months to feel right again, but I'm

*glad that I did it myself. It means that if it comes again I can take it in
my stride.*

Her strategies and those described above represent only a part
of a wide range of self-help approaches to anxiety, but they are by
far the simplest and the most effective to tackle on your own. The
books on stress listed under Chapter 3 at the end of the book go in
more detail into the wide variety of things that you can do to help
yourself.

Psychological therapies

If you approach your general practitioners about your anxiety –
and most people will do this because of the physical nature of
many of the symptoms – they may treat you themselves with rest,
understanding and possibly an anti-anxiety drug, or they may
refer you to a psychologist or a psychiatrist. The latter may also
prescribe drugs or may in turn refer you on to a psychologist, since
their methods are generally regarded as particularly useful for
anxiety states.

Which type of therapy the clinical psychologist uses will
depend on their orientation (see Chapter 2), but one of the most
common comes under the general heading of behaviour therapy.
The underlying theory to this is that over time we all learn
certain responses to certain situations, one response being fear.
Just as these can be learned, so too they can be unlearned. Thus
one of their basic strategies is to teach people to use relaxation in
order to learn to associate relaxation rather than fear with certain
situations. As people come to realise that they can control their
anxiety themselves, their more general fear diminishes and confidence begins to return.

The therapy may also include filling in daily diaries in order to
discover which situations are easy and which are difficult and also
to try to discover whether there are any consequences of the
anxious behaviour. For example, it may be that someone close,
like a spouse, only seems to care when you feel panicky. In this
case it will be important to ask him or her for caring at other times,
so that eliminating the anxiety symptoms doesn't mean an end to
loving attention.

Another approach is that of cognitive-behavioural therapy

which is used to help people to discover the negative thoughts that precede the anxiety: thoughts such as, 'I'll never manage to get it right', or 'They'll think I'm an idiot', or 'I'll never get better'. The therapy aims to show what a powerful effect these thoughts have on our symptoms and our behaviour, and teaches ways to challenge them and to substitute more useful thoughts. Although this approach is more often used for depression rather than anxiety, it is an extremely useful part of treatment for panic. Salkovskis and Clark have had excellent results by using their over-breathing model (p. 47) to explain the patients' symptoms (that is, providing them with a more acceptable reason for their problems), and also by teaching them to slow their breathing and reduce their oxygen intake. Just as the self-help methods aim to do, these behavioural approaches are designed to help you gain control over your life once again.

When Stephen finally agreed with his wife that it was time he received professional help, his general practitioner asked him to see the clinical psychologist who had recently begun to work in the practice. At first they met each week for an hour, and later the appointments became shorter and more spaced. During the first few sessions, they worked together to try to understand what the responsibility of the new job meant to Stephen, since it seemed to be a central issue in his anxiety and panic attacks. Stephen realised gradually that he had always felt responsible for people, often when there was little that he could actually do about their situation. His mother had been depressed for much of his childhood, and he had gradually turned himself into the family clown as a way to try to make things better. Since a child can never successfully take on responsibility for a parent's happiness (though many try to do so), the attempt was doomed to failure, and it was this sense of failure that haunted Stephen when he took on real responsibility at the mine.

This insight into his problems may not have been an essential part of Stephen's recovery, but he felt it a relief to have some understanding, and began to notice when he took responsibility inappropriately for aspects of other people's lives, such as his wife's. He realised too that he was seeing responsibility at work as stretching far beyond reasonable safety towards keeping his men happy, involving himself in their personal difficulties and so on.

During this period he learnt a method of relaxation and began making excursions further and further from home. He also learnt to challenge thoughts like 'I'll have a panic attack if I do that', and 'Nothing this simple can possibly help me', and 'Everyone at work will laugh at me when I go back.' After a couple of months his psychologist accompanied him and drove to the mine, and they walked around the site together. She waited in the car while he talked to his boss about a date for his return, and he was delighted to discover how sympathetic this man could be. He learnt ways to keep up his progress on his own, and what to do when things went wrong, and six months later came to tell her how good things were.

I can actually look back on the whole experience positively now. I really feel I've gained something by going through it and by altering my life in useful ways. If it hadn't happened I might have had a heart attack by now, I was worrying so much about everything and everyone. My wife's happier too; she says I don't keep fussing round her and let her be more independent.

In other more exploratory forms of psychotherapy, there will be less structure and advice and few or no tasks set for you to achieve. In these therapies, you and your helper will try together to understand your feelings now, and the way these may relate to other relationships both in the present and in the past. In this way you can gain insight into how you operate towards the world, and so change aspects of yourself that don't seem to be helping. Stephen's psychologist used these methods in their first meetings. She noticed early on how he always asked how she was, commented that she looked tired or cold, and worried that he was boring her; in other words, he was taking responsibility for her in whatever way he could, despite the fact that he was supposed to be there to be helped. By pointing out how he behaved towards her, she was able to guess how he might be towards other people.

Sarah's anxiety was really quite severe, very mixed with depression. In fact, suspecting she was going mad, she went to a general practitioner, and he gave her some tranquillisers and told her that lots of women felt like that. She only took a few before deciding that they did little but add a woolly head to her other feelings.

But something did change for her. Perhaps his low-key approach was useful, perhaps talking to her friend at work, perhaps the fact that they moved to a rural part of England, and she was forced to be active: whatever it was, she gradually realised she wanted to get better and began looking after herself in simple ways. She spent hours digging a garden, and went for long walks every day. She liked the locals and began to enjoy making friends. The dreadful physical symptoms faded on their own and with them went the thoughts of sin and punishment. Years later, however, when her marriage was getting rocky, she went to a counsellor who used gestalt therapy involving talking to an empty chair (see p. 13). In her mind she put her husband in the chair, and began to tell him how hurt she felt by various aspects of their marriage.

> *Gradually I found myself becoming more and more angry, and it was all to do with the very beginning of our relationship. I was roaring at him, telling him what I felt about him refusing to go to Canada so I lost my career and family and everything. I couldn't believe just how angry I was. I banged away at the chair, crying and shouting. So much rage! After that our whole relationship changed for the better. It was as though I could now allow myself to love him and appreciate him fully for the first time. It explained so much about my earlier breakdown: all that anger swallowed down had to do something to me, that's for sure. No wonder I was shaking all over, my heart was crashing, and I had to keep racing to the loo – I was exploding with it. I listen to my body now: I find it tells me things quite clearly!*

Drug treatment

Matthew began taking tranquillisers to decrease the symptoms of jet-lag. He had to travel between London and the States every couple of weeks, despite still finding flying quite frightening. The rest of his life he did little more than work which filled most of his waking hours. The jet-lag was creating quite serious difficulties in his concentration, he thought, and drugs might let him regulate his sleep, and so work more efficiently. He found them useful for this and decided to take them when he was actually flying as well, because they seemed to take away his old fears. Then he used them too for meetings at home simply because he found he worried about not taking them: something might happen. Gradually they became a regular part of his life and he found he needed to raise the dose and then to change the brand in order not to suffer various symptoms such as shaking hands and a dreadful sensitivity to noise.

I think I'd have carried on taking more and more for ever. I had no wife any longer to tell me to cut down, and I certainly didn't let male friends know what I was taking. The crunch came when I began to get really sloppy about my work and irritable with people. A new doctor in the practice told me I should give them up as quickly as possible, and put me on a regime of cutting my daily dose by one tablet each week. I had to take a couple of weeks off work at the beginning because I had some quite frightening physical symptoms. And I just couldn't face flying at all then. My company were good, though. They were used to seeing people with alcohol problems but not tranquillisers! But they sent me to a good bloke who taught me how to relax without drugs. I'm fine now, but looking back, it all seemed so unnecessary.

Most of the drugs prescribed for anxiety are the 'minor' tranquillisers which come under the general heading of the benzodiazepines. The most commonly prescribed are Valium (diazepam), Librium (chlordiazepoxide), Ativan (lorazepam), and Mogadon (nitrazepam), used mainly for sleep problems. Side-effects include lethargy, 'hangover' symptoms, coordination problems, sexual difficulties, memory loss, and confusion in the elderly. However, it should be remembered that side-effects are extremely idiosyncratic: although these are the ones most commonly seen, individuals may experience others quite unique to them, so no list can be exhaustive.

These drugs were developed in the late fifties and their prescription rose dramatically throughout the sixties and seventies when it began to be recognised that their use was out of all proportion to their need and that long-term use posed a serious addiction problem. By 1977 it was reported that 45 million prescriptions a year were being given, almost a fifth of all drugs prescribed. As publicity about their effects became more widespread this figure dropped to 29 million in 1981, but despite numerous warning articles, they are still heavily prescribed not only for anxiety but also for sleep problems, life stresses, and a whole range of physical illnesses for which the doctor suspects there is a psychological cause – illnesses such as spastic colon, rashes, menstrual difficulties, backache, migraine, and so on. The 'That's Life!' programme on BBC Television conducted a survey in 1984 and found almost a quarter of the population of the United Kingdom had taken a tranquilliser at some time, and a quarter of those for periods of one to 15 years.

Women are far more likely to be prescribed these drugs than men, perhaps for a number of reasons: they tend to visit their doctors more than men; they are more likely to present their problems in psychological terms and admit to unhappiness and difficulties in their lives, while men are more likely to insist on seeing problems as physical; and women are less likely to use alcohol to temporarily relieve their problems. Thus in the 'That's Life!'/MORI poll, four times as many women as men were prescribed one of the minor tranquillisers including one in three women between the ages of 45 to 59!

Initially, the benzodiazepines reduce feelings of anxiety, relax tense muscles, induce sleepiness; a low dose taken for a short period of time (preferably less than four weeks) may allow people to feel calm enough to take some necessary action over crises in their lives. However, prolonged anxiety is not a crisis, and its effects may continue for much longer than those associated with life stress. If you are taking any version of these drugs you must realise clearly that they only deal with the symptoms of anxiety, they do not treat the problem underlying it; and that their capacity to relieve the symptoms decreases over time. This means that your dose must increase or the make of drug must change in order to get the same amount of relief. In addition, various reports show that, after a while, it is possible that they may make you *more* irritable and even aggressive, more anxious and depressed, and actually make you sleep *less* well. In elderly people they may cause confusion and incontinence.

If you are taking any of the so-called 'minor' tranquillisers, remember that driving is just as dangerous as it would be with an excess of alcohol, especially on motorways, and, since reaction times are slowed down, they are likely to have potentially dangerous effects if you take part in hazardous activities either at work or in the home. They should also be avoided during pregnancy and breastfeeding, and not taken in conjunction with alcohol, tea, coffee, anti-histamines, and a number of other drugs. Make sure your doctor, or the hospital, is very aware of any drugs you are taking.

Because the benzodiazepines don't actually cure anything, your anxiety symptoms are likely to return as soon as you stop taking the drug: there is still controversy about whether these are withdrawal symptoms or the original anxiety returning. Once again, this very much depends upon the individual, and there is no way of predicting how stopping their use will affect you. The symptoms of withdrawal may include any of the following: strange metallic tastes in your mouth; confusion; difficulty in speaking; blurred vision; heightened sensitivity; and burning sensations around your face and head.

Because of the risk of withdrawal symptoms and a return of the anxiety itself, there are two rules to note when you decide to give up benzodiazepines. First, use the self-help and behavioural techniques in the previous section for at least two weeks before you begin. You may find your doctor knows of a group that you can join in order to make the whole procedure more comfortable, and these certainly provide support when times are difficult, and are very effective. Tranx, the National Tranquilliser Advisory Council, will give you support by phone or information about their groups, as will your local MIND. Second, cut down quite slowly, especially if you are on a large daily dose. Dr Vernon Coleman, in his book *Life Without Tranquillisers*, suggests that you should cut your dose in half every fortnight until you can no longer do so. However, if you are on a large dose (such as six tablets a day), decrease them by one daily tablet each week. The rate at which you come off these drugs will depend on what else is happening in your life and how much support you have from friends or family or a group.

Other drugs prescribed may include an antidepressant and anti-anxiety drug together, while others, like Stelazine, are much more powerful and would only be used in cases of severe anxiety. Occasionally your doctor might prescribe a drug which can relieve a specific symptom, such as beta-blockers for an irregular or racing heart. It might be worth suggesting to him or her that you wish to try some of the self-help strategies before beginning such drugs unless they are considered really essential, or at least try the self-help alongside the medicines.

Hospitalisation

Very rarely anxiety builds up to such an intensity, often with considerable speed, that relatives, friends and the doctor concerned decide that the sufferer needs the protection of hospital.

Janet had been feeling tense and somewhat depressed ever since they'd moved from Scotland the previous year. Her husband's promotion made the change necessary, she appreciated that; but it meant she lost close contact with her parents and with good friends that she had known since childhood, friends who accepted her for what she was. Ben's new job meant that their social life now revolved around his colleagues, clever men and women with whom Janet felt inferior, and more and more alone and afraid. She decided to concentrate on her children, but they were now in their teens and growing so fast that the eldest two were already considerably bigger than her. Sometimes, walking into her kitchen and finding them sitting round the table with their huge friends, for a moment she would fail to recognise them at all, and would find herself seized with terror at their presence. At night, when they were asleep, the terror often continued and, thinking of them more easily as little children, she would spend hours checking that they were tucked in warm, that the windows were secure, and that they were breathing properly.

This behaviour escalated so that she was rarely sleeping or eating, and shadows were turned into horrors lurking to harm her and her family. The underlying fear that her world was being turned upside down by the move was being given a reality in the bizarre way her eyes were playing tricks. Her husband and her doctor decided she needed more help than they could provide, and took her into hospital. She was given Largactil (chlorpromazine), which is one of the so-called major tranquillisers given in cases of schizophrenia (see Chapter 13) and gradually became calmer over the next two weeks, and began to sleep and eat a little. She was discharged and, with the help of benzodiazepines, managed to cope adequately at home for a few months before the whole thing started again. This time she was admitted to a different hospital, and a young woman psychiatrist, beginning to train in psychotherapy, began to see her regularly. Their sessions allowed Janet to get a glimpse of her anger at what had happened to her life, and she began to recognise aspects of her strength again.

Looking back, I think I needed the hospital. Well, not necessarily a hospital, but a place away from the family where I could grow a bit again. The first time I went in was quite useless, because nothing was done to change things, but I got a lot out of the other place, especially my talks with Angela. She left because she was being moved around different hospitals, but when I was discharged I approached our local women's therapy service, and saw someone there for six months or so. I feel now I've been on some long quest, but it's been worth it. It's let me feel independent from both Ben and the children without being scared about it.

Such a severe case of anxiety is quite rare and very frightening for those concerned. Nevertheless, it does show how help can come from a number of sources. It shows too that it sometimes pays to 'shop around', and that recovery even in such cases is still very possible.

Chapter

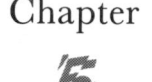

Phobias

Michael sat there looking tense and glancing suspiciously towards the corners of the room. At 21, blonde and burly, he was a picture of muscular masculinity. He'd just managed to find a job as a warehouseman in a tinned food factory, but after only a week he reported as sick. They'd given him one more chance. It was a pattern that had repeated itself often since he left school. His father, at the end of his tether, had sent him for help. With great reluctance, he finally described his constant fear of spiders.

I've always been terrified of them, for as long as I can remember. At school it meant that I could only play in certain parts of the yard, and that I would make sure I didn't get chosen to help with the PE gear or get the stuff out from under the stage. But on the whole, when I was young it didn't seem so hard to handle, except that kids would find out and tease me and I'd often get into fights or have to change friends. But jobs are a nightmare. My first one was an apprentice plumber. I was really pleased with myself. But within the first couple of days I realised it was going to be completely impossible: I couldn't put my hand under any floorboards; I couldn't even go down into cellars. I was totally terrified but I couldn't tell anyone why. It seemed so stupid. I felt ill every time I even thought of what I might have to do that day and so after a fortnight I went off sick, and never actually went back.

My next job was as a labourer, but that also ended within days when I picked up a rock, saw a spider, and promptly dropped the rock on my foot and broke some small bones. I stayed unemployed for ages after that, till Dad got me the warehouseman's job. I thought canned food stores would be OK, and I haven't actually seen a spider, but I can't bring myself to do things like count the boxes at the back of the store, or anything like that. I can't think of any job really where I would feel completely safe!

Michael was, of course, suffering from a phobia – an intense irrational fear of some object or situation. The sight or the thought of the object, or anything similar to it brings on severe anxiety symptoms and even full-blown panic attacks (see Chapter 4). How serious these symptoms are will depend on how closely related a particular object is to the one most feared. So a person whose greatest fear concerns large black dogs may well experience only a mild flurry of symptoms when confronted with a drawing of a small poodle, but a full panic attack as a black labrador hurls himself through the door to greet him.

Compared to those suffering from general anxiety states, people with phobias alone are comparatively rare. Most of us know the names of those most common: claustrophobia (a fear of confined spaces); acrophobia (fear of heights); hydrophobia (fear of water), and so on. But we can come to fear almost any specific thing that exists in the world: some individuals will suffer phobias concerning birds, spiders, thunder, the dark, dolls, scissors, cats, telephones, wolves, sealed letters, aeroplanes, and so on. Agoraphobia, traditionally defined as a fear of open spaces, will be discussed in a separate section after the more specific objects of fear.

This is perhaps the psychological problem most easily tolerated by the public at large. It has little stigma attached to it and is most usually treated by both family and friends as somewhat amusing – something not to be taken seriously, and even the means of providing ammunition for practical jokes. Part of this attitude undoubtedly stems from the fact that those who suffer from phobias have usually done so in some form or other since they were very young, and over the years have adjusted their lives in some way in order to avoid the object that might provoke the symptoms. It lacks, therefore, the drama of 'real' nervous breakdowns, but its consequences can be equally distressing.

It's clear, however, that many people find that they are not too incapacitated by their phobias. For example, someone with a fear of flying may find it a nuisance at times, but a full rich life can be led without ever going near an airport. If the sufferer does require to travel, even long distances can be achieved by all sorts of means of transport: both the QE2 and the smallest cargo ship will usually hold passengers not only seeking luxury or adventure, but also simply too frightened to fly. On the other hand, a fear of thunder will usually mean having to pay constant attention to weather forecasts, and a refusal to leave the house on days that even hint of storms. A severe fear of birds may leave a person housebound for years.

Like all other forms of psychological problems, no one can say exactly how phobias arise. There is no doubt that some fairly specific ones can come about by a frightening early experience such as happened to Emma on her third birthday.

Her parents organised a puppet show of Little Red Riding Hood at her birthday party, making and operating the puppets themselves. It was very successful and at the end of it the mother came out and was laughing and chatting with the children. Suddenly the wolf popped his head up from where he'd been lying since his violent end: 'Is there a little girl called Emma here?' he asked. Emma walked up towards the makeshift theatre and gazed at the wolf. 'Me,' she whispered. 'Then I'm going to eat you up,' roared the wolf.

Emma screamed and her father appeared holding the puppet and laughing. It was clear that all his attempted reassurance did not quite convince his daughter. From then on Emma, without involving her parents, would take anything up to an hour painstakingly searching her room for possible wolves before she went to bed, but nothing quite convinced her of their absence and she often suffered nightmares where they swallowed her whole.

But the origins of most phobias are more difficult to establish. It may be that people are actually suffering from anxiety, as we described in the previous chapter, and then in some way 'choose' an object to make sense of their frightening symptoms: it's often harder to feel afraid without apparent reason, than to be able to explain your anxieties in terms of one particular object or situation. A similar switch can occur with intense worrying: 'I'm such a worrier,' a man will say. 'If I haven't got something to worry about, I'll find something.' What he means is, he feels constantly anxious and needs to give his anxiety some understandable cause.

Therapists who work more along Freudian lines, might see a phobia as symbolic of some deeper fear; for example, a fear of confined spaces might deep down concern a fear of being smothered, trapped, or tightly restricted in some way, probably by a parent. Once again, while it might in some circumstances feel reassuring to understand the cause of a symptom, what matters most is that things change, and the majority of phobias can be relieved relatively easily.

WHAT CAN BE DONE?

As with most psychological problems, phobias can fade with time or, more accurately, with good experiences that provide evidence to contradict your fear. For example, although someone with a phobia of dogs may not make friends with anyone who has a dog, if close friends decide to get one he or she is all at once forced to make a choice between confronting the pet or giving up the friends. Depending upon the strength of the phobia and the size and apparent ferocity of the dog, many adults will decide that now's the time to do something about their fear.

Like all fears, confrontation is ultimately the only remedy; all the other methods, like drugs or relaxation, are prescribed only in order to make the confrontation easier. With friends to help make the meeting less of an ordeal, there is every chance of success. However, it really is important that the first time this happens the animal (or whatever else you're tackling) is relatively well behaved and docile. If this is unlikely, then set yourself a hierarchy of dogs belonging to people you know, and choose the least fearful to confront first. Your aim is to have a safe relaxed atmosphere that will allow you to approach animals that hold progressively more fear.

Before exposing yourself to something that you've been afraid of for so many years, it might seem a good idea to have a strong drink first. It isn't. Alcohol is quite likely to let you be more relaxed and carefree, that's true. But the problem is that the aim of the experience is to help you to unlearn your fear – to learn that you can pat a dog without your worst fantasies taking place – and what you learn under the influence of alcohol does not carry over very well into the sober state (Chapter 10). So you would still have to unlearn your fear while you're sober.

Occasionally people report other ways that have helped. For example, Emma kept her fear of wolves until she was ten. Although she knew it was irrational – there were no longer wolves in Britain – she continued to search under her bed each night, found stories featuring wolves less than entertaining, and still had nightmares about them several times a month. Her parents' taking her to the zoo to show her what small, thin, pathetic animals wolves were in real life had done nothing to allay her fears. One night, however, she began dreaming the same old nightmare. The wolves were coming along the corridor towards her bedroom door. She knew that they would snuffle around outside for a while till they smelt her, then rush into the bedroom and swallow her whole. They'd done it so many times before.

In my dream I remember suddenly deciding enough was enough. If I was going to be eaten yet again, I'd put up a fight this time. So I leapt out of bed and met the wolves face to face at the top of the stairs. They looked a bit shocked! I took the first by the throat and then the second and hurled each of them down the stairs. My strength was really fantastic and it felt marvellously easy. I can still remember the feeling. They lay in a crumpled pile of mangy fur at the bottom of the staircase and, in my dream, I remember walking back to bed feeling ten foot tall. I never feared wolves again. It was quite extraordinary.

We can't all have such convenient dreams, and many of us will have phobias about objects which are difficult to control; for example thunder, or birds. If your phobia means you find it necessary to alter aspects of your life in inconvenient ways, and if you've tried to help yourself and not succeeded; if it concerns things that are not so easy to confront, or not so predictable in their actions, then it may be a good idea to seek professional help of some kind.

Psychological Therapies

By far the most commonly used and effective treatment for phobias is behaviour therapy (see Chapter 2). The most traditional form involves setting up a hierarchy of feared objects and using relaxation to control the anxiety provoked by each, starting with the one that causes the least problems and working up towards the top. Although this is clearly something that you could do yourself, and self-help techniques are all based upon this treatment from clinical psychology, it really makes a great difference having the support and encouragement of someone that you trust while you carry out tasks that have been difficult for so long.

Michael's psychologist helped him to draw up a hierarchy of spiders, ranging from tiny money spiders at the bottom to large hairy ones with long legs at the top. He was taught relaxation and began to use it to travel up the list, at first represented only by photographs. He found he could handle this fairly easily and also could hold various realistic models with a minimum of fear. He then began with real spiders and found that money spiders presented no problem and he could let them stay in his hand. The next stop up was a house spider, about an inch across.

My psychologist held the glass jar up for me to see, and then handed it to me. I could feel the panic symptoms starting, but I knew it couldn't get out and I used the relaxation quite successfully. When I said I was OK, we went to the sink and she put the plug in and tipped in the spider. She let it crawl across her finger a couple of times to show me it was all right, and then she asked me to see how close I could get to touching it. I was doing real well and getting to within an inch of it. I felt anxious, but nothing I couldn't control. Finally, she made me lay my hand palm down in the sink and encouraged the spider to run across it. She wouldn't let me pull my hand away, and that felt like a turning point. I found after that I could touch it quite easily, and even let her drop it onto my hand and my knees – something I'd always been terrified of happening.

Between them, they worked their way a little higher up the list before agreeing that holding large spiders or poking your finger at tarantulas was not particularly useful, and they'd gone far enough. Most importantly, to end they had a couple of sessions where Michael was asked to put his hand into the backs of dark cupboards, and under wardrobes and floorboards. He used relaxation as well as phrases he'd found helpful (for example, 'I know I can do it'; 'I've done more daring things than this') to counteract any negative thoughts that preceded feelings of panic. Finding he was now able to work without any real problems enlarged his confidence dramatically.

Very occasionally, where one phobia ends and you leave therapy, another begins, which is what you might expect if, for example, the specific phobia was really a narrowing of some wider anxiety. In this case the therapist would want to treat your anxiety more generally and may want to consider what it is about your relationship together that allows you to stop being afraid while you're seeing each other. In this way it may, for example, be possible to build such a supportive relationship into the rest of your life.

It is often necessary to take a more exploratory approach to a phobia for other reasons. For example, it's difficult to treat a fear of thunder with a hierarchy. Mary, suffering from this phobia for as long as she could remember, described hiding under the bed for hours as a child. Her mother, busy with seven other children, had apparently never noticed. Asked by her doctor what her husband did now when she was afraid, she admitted that she never let him know if she could help it – she still took herself off somewhere to hide – and they'd certainly never talked about it. It was suggested to her that she seemed to be acting as she did as a child, presuming that no one would comfort her. She agreed to discuss the whole thing with her husband and to ask him for his help next time she felt afraid.

> *I found he really wanted to help me. He'd felt really inadequate when he knew I was in a state but I never asked him for help. I still feel afraid of thunder, but it really is getting better. I'm starting to think that what was most frightening was the loneliness of suffering on my own, rather than the thunder itself.*

Drug treatment

As in cases of general anxiety, any of the minor tranquillisers may be used to reduce the symptoms, though all the provisos about their limited use, addictive qualities and side-effects inevitably apply (pp. 54–56). Occasionally they are used as a way of confronting the feared object, either where it cannot be avoided (like going to the dentist), or alongside behaviour therapy in an early part of treatment. However, just as with the use of alcohol, it is your brain free from drugs that needs to learn there is nothing to fear, and the use of tranquillisers will rarely provide a short cut.

Other treatments

Once again, no one method can claim total success, and more alternative therapists such as hypnotists may well provide relief for some people, though the numbers of people setting themselves up as experts in this field is a cause for concern. At the other extreme, short-term hospitalisation, though extremely rare for phobias, may allow you the chance to have intense behavioural treatment where your fear is really affecting most aspects of your life.

AGORAPHOBIA

Agoraphobia is by far the commonest form of phobia, and also potentially the most serious since people who suffer it – and at least three quarters are women – may eventually fear leaving the house at all, or even staying in alone. The name comes from the Greek and means 'fear of the market place' but in the last century it was used mainly to describe a condition where people become severely anxious when confronted by open spaces. Today it is used quite generally to describe any fear of the world outside of home, from supermarkets to the moors; from theatres to long empty corridors. The boundary between this and an anxiety state is by no means distinct, and the case of Stephen (described in Chapter 4) would equally well be seen as a classic example of agoraphobia.

Like Stephen, the problem often begins with a panic attack which is followed by dizziness and other symptoms of anxiety whenever a similar situation is faced, or even thought about. People suffering from this problem report being afraid they will faint in the theatre in front of everyone, that they will die alone on the moors, or perhaps that they will do something unspeakable in public. As in cases of general anxiety, what these people are actually suffering from is a fear of fear itself: they are terrified of *feeling* the dizziness, the palpitations, the awful nausea which are in fact the symptoms of being very afraid. Many worry constantly about what is happening in their bodies and many, not surprisingly, become depressed. Heather describes her experiences:

> *I know precisely when it started. I was at a meeting of Young Wives at our local church. I'd only been a couple of times before because we'd not long been in the district. And I let out a rude noise. You know, broke wind. I thought I would die with embarrassment. I was shaking all over but I got myself out of the hall and ran all the way home. I was crying and in a dreadful state. I know it sounds daft, and I wonder sometimes if I'm not going mad, but I just daren't leave the house now. I've not been out since unless it's dark, and then I just run to the dustbin or something.*

Certainly not everyone with the problem of agoraphobia is housebound. Many struggle on, feeling constantly apprehensive while outside but managing to hold down jobs or do the shopping, at least in the corner shop if not the supermarket. Sometimes they will find something that makes the fear more tolerable; for example, if their spouse or a relative accompanies them, or if they wear dark glasses (as if the possibility of being recognised brings on the fear), or having a drink before they go. Others will always sit downstairs near the door of the bus, or at the end of the aisle nearest an exit in the cinema, so they know they can leave should the panic appear. Although these are all personal strategies to reduce the fear and allow the person to enjoy a fuller life, if you notice yourself or someone close to you altering their behaviour in any of these ways, it would be advisable to consider help, either self-help or from a professional. Like all psychological difficulties, catching the symptoms before they get hard to control makes a cure so much easier. But people are also often good at covering up the problem. At the end of the miners' strike in 1985, Marsha Marshall was interviewed about the part she had played in fund-raising and about the agoraphobia she had had to conquer: 'An agoraphobic', Marsha told her interviewer, 'makes a good liar. You're never in. You've just this minute gone out.'*

Although some people do manage to hold down very demanding jobs despite suffering the symptoms of agoraphobia, it may also be the case that having the job provides a demand which actually

---

* Aitken, S. (1985). The case of the agoraphobic miner's wife. *Changes, 3,* 110.

stops the problem becoming too severe. Thus unemployment, whether voluntary or otherwise, may stop people confronting their tolerable fears each day, and this may quite quickly allow things to become out of control.

Without demands of some sort placed upon them people who have experienced some anxiety away from home can easily slip into being housebound and dependent. The first patient I ever saw when I was training to be a clinical psychologist was Enid. Nine years previously she had left a well-paid job as a personal assistant to the manager of a large organisation in order to look after her ailing mother. When her mother died, she felt nervous at the thought of seeking new employment and, supported by her husband, she stayed at home. She gradually found going out alone more and more difficult and her husband did more and more to help and her anxiety grew. When I was asked to see her she had not left the house, even to hang washing on the line, for four years apart from occasional trips after dark accompanying her husband while he shopped.

I had intended to visit her in her home, but became quite lost and so rang her from the nearest village and asked if she would mind meeting me in the coffee shop. This was no daring strategy on my part; simply a useful ignorance of the real meaning of her condition. But she caught her first bus for five years and met me within half an hour. She felt dreadfully anxious, of course, but as we chatted about what had been happening to her, she found the symptoms subsiding just a little. Realising I had placed the first demands on her for some years, I decided not to drive her home and let her catch the bus again. It was no miracle cure and I continued to see her weekly over the next six months, but she always came to my workplace, initially with her husband, and finally alone.

What causes it?

Like other phobias and some anxiety states, agoraphobia often starts with a panic attack and develops by a fear of its repetition. However, with such a preponderance of women, especially around the ages of 25–35, researchers have been wondering if there isn't sometimes another factor in the cause. Many women suffering from agoraphobia have very caring, helpful husbands upon whom they have become more and more dependent. Therapists have noticed that, if the woman improves with treatment, occasionally these husbands will become depressed or anxious themselves; sometimes they insist that treatment is ended as it's obviously forcing their wives to do too much; others might become almost jealous of the therapists. It seems that, for these couples, the agoraphobia is playing some necessary part in the marriage, and so it is important to look to some aspect of the relationship for a cause. This of course will have implications for treatment.

What can be done?

The treatments for agoraphobia are basically the same as those for general anxiety or for more specific phobias, described in the preceding chapter and above. Thus the majority will use relaxation and a hierarchy of feared situations and practise confronting them both in the imagination and in real life. Occasionally, a procedure called flooding might be used where, perhaps alone or along with three or four people with similar problems, you might be asked by your therapist to stay in the feared situation for three or four hours, or at least until you are able to do so reasonably comfortably. Whether it's done all at once, as in flooding, or more slowly using the hierarchy (systematic desensitisation), the important element in all the treatments is exposure to what makes you afraid. Knowing that you've faced it and survived without any of the terrible things happening that you'd imagined so often, lets you face it each time with less and less fear and so your confidence grows.

However, since it was noticed that people who had become very dependent upon their spouses prior to therapy frequently relapsed despite having completely controlled their fear, many therapists now insist that both parties to the marriage attend sessions together, at least for a few sessions. Enid made great progress after meeting me in the coffee shop and seemed to be actually enjoying coming for her appointments. Her husband sat and waited for her in the car outside. One day just as she'd left my office I noticed him standing on the opposite pavement, staring up at my window. My secretary said he had been there all through the session. The next week Enid cancelled her appointment just at the last minute. She told me she was full of dreadful aches and pains and her husband thought that all this travelling to and fro each week was bad for her. I suggested that she bring him next time and then I could explain just what we were doing.

He soon became interested and involved in her progress and things went fine again for a few weeks but then, as she began to do her own shopping, she told me he was becoming very morose and irritable. I saw them again as a couple and we started at last to talk about his jealousy of Enid that he found so hard to control. He was frightened that, if she got really well and started to work again, she might meet someone she fancied more than him and he would be alone. They both admitted too, that they had always had problems with their sexual relationship, and that made worse his fear of her infidelity. So, kept like a bird in a gilded cage, she was well cared for but imprisoned by the man whose fear was probably equal to her own. They received sex therapy and some brief marital therapy and from then on her progress was assured.

Certainly not all people who suffer from agoraphobia will have such difficulties in their marriage, but clearly a lack of demands placed upon them will usually mean that nothing will change – at least not for the better! Of course, the therapist makes demands, but life can do so too, as the case of Marsha Marshall illustrates so well. Having suffered agoraphobia for some years, dependent on her husband at home and alcohol to go out, the miners' strike began and her husband was arrested.

> *Police rang me and said that he'd been arrested, but they couldn't tell me what for. So I said I'm going down t'strike centre to find out. But you see, strike centre was a pub. I did have a drink, but I didn't need it. And I'm sat there saying 'If I could do this, if I could do that.'*
>
> *Next thing I were asked to go on television. I said 'Oh, Christ, no I can't go on telly', and then I just says, 'Yes, I will go.' It had to be done so quick because they rang me at half eleven. It weren't easy I can tell you.*

As the interviewer says, 'Marsha appeared on a national TV network, putting the case for the miners' strike, talking to millions of viewers, where a day before she avoided talking to anyone except her family.'

Within weeks she was raising funds around Britain and abroad, addressing thousands from the platform and marching at the head of rallies. Looking back at the strike and the challenge that it provided her with, Marsha says: 'It were the finest thing – it's a shame to say it wi' so much suffering and hardship – but it were the finest thing that ever happened to me.'

Chapter

Depression

Most people know when they're depressed. They recognise the feelings of sadness or apathy that last not just hours or days, but months or even years. They recognise too the difficulty in enjoying anything any more, and the tears that well up unexpectedly not only when they talk about themselves, but also when someone shows they care, or even over countless events on television, both sad and joyful. The sadness may be constant, or it may come and go with little apparent reason. While some will let people know the way they feel, others will go to great lengths to hide it, feeling it simply confirms their views about themselves as weak and useless.

Linda beamed as she walked into the office and shook hands. She was tall and very smartly dressed. Her makeup was perfect and while she smiled her eyes flashed me warm, engaging looks. But, of course, she was tense; most people would be, coming to see a psychologist for the first time. I suggested that it might seem a bit strange coming here, asking for help. Instantly her eyes filled with tears and her voice choked, as she carried on laughing, talking and sobbing all at the same time.

'That must be real agony,' I said. 'Trying to make me feel things are fine by laughing, and trying to fight back all that misery at the same time. You are allowed to feel wretched, you know.'

At this, she turned her head slightly away from me, and the tears flowed more freely, though she still flashed the odd rueful smile between sobs. After a few minutes she blew her nose, wiped the mascara carefully from beneath her eyes, and laughed: 'Aren't I stupid?' she said.

Linda illustrates just one aspect of the many men and women who come, or who are sent, for help for their depression. She was the clown with the mask depicting a smiling face, while inside she wept constantly. She was in conflict between longing for someone to take care of her – and thinking that if she showed her need and her distress, she would be thought weak, stupid, would be taken advantage of and tricked. Moreover, it became clear that she didn't feel she deserved anyone's help or caring: she had no right to feel depressed with a good job as a personal assistant, and a man who seemed to want to be with her (though she found it impossible to believe), and somewhere to live. She shouldn't be depressed and, more fundamentally, she didn't deserve any help because deep down she was nasty, bad and hateful: not worth loving or caring for by anyone.

People describe their depressed feelings in a variety of ways: they will often see it as an emptiness within them, almost a physical hollowness. Some may take this for depression, while others may fill the emptiness with alcohol, or vast quantities of food or, symbolically, by spending money. Others describe their feelings as an intense heaviness pulling them down or crushing them from every side. In her excellent book, *Depression: The Way Out of Your Prison*, Dorothy Rowe tells how she asks clients, 'If you could paint a picture of what you are feeling, what sort of picture would you paint?' The images she gets are of being alone in a fog or an empty wasteland, crawling on and on to an empty horizon, in an endless tunnel, or compressed in a large black balloon. The person is trapped in some way, and always terribly alone. Linda described her depression like this:

I'm hanging on to the edge of a ghastly bottomless pit, knowing that at any moment I may drop down into it. Actually, it can't be totally bottomless because I know it contains vile sludge and unimaginable horrors. I seem to have been hanging here for so long and I'm dreadfully exhausted.

Apart from the primary sign of this deep, painful sadness and loneliness, people who are depressed are often filled with intense self-dislike. You see yourself, even if you are extremely successful, as really simply fooling people: about your abilities, your charm, your strength, and so on. You live on the edge of terror that you'll be found out, exposed, and (if you were pushed far enough to think about the consequences of all this) ultimately ridiculed.

Akin to this lack of self-esteem depressed people will usually blame themselves for all the things that go wrong around them, and also for the psychological problems they're enduring. No wonder they don't think they deserve help! They find it equally difficult to take the credit for the good things that happen, or for the positive moves they make: 'I never do anything useful,' said Linda. 'You came here,' I suggested. 'Only because my GP made me,' she sighed.

Apart from these problems of lowered self-esteem, if you have depression you can see no end to the misery you're experiencing. It is this hopelessness and worthlessness that makes suicide seem a rational act for some depressed people. If you can see no hope of change, you often have to be sent for help rather than seeking it for yourself (apart from the fact you feel you don't deserve it!), but this is sometimes considerably relieved at the first consultation by having the possibilities for change spelt out. That first gleam of hope is the beginning of the road to recovery.

There are physical signs as well. Whereas mild feelings of depression may make you eat and eat, if these become more serious there is a definite loss of appetite. People suffering from anxiety may have trouble getting off to sleep, but those with depression find they wake much earlier than usual, and that those hours of early dawn are sometimes the worst in the day. They tell of their constant exhaustion, that they've lost all interest in sex (though in the early stages sex, like food, may be a frequent source of comfort), and that they have memory problems and great difficulty concentrating and making decisions.

There is always a sense of apathy, pointlessness and deadness which can be the most exasperating aspect for those near to someone who is depressed. For some people this deadness is the primary symptom, taking away even sadness. In Judith Guest's novel, *Ordinary People*, one of her characters describes this: '. . . depression is not sobbing and crying and giving vent, it is plain and simple reduction of feeling. Reduction, see? Of all feeling. People who keep stiff upper lips find that it's damn hard to smile.'

At its worst depression can stop all movement, and people retreat into themselves totally, not communicating at all and often not moving from their beds for any reason.

Manic-depression is discussed in Chapter 14. In this disorder the mood fluctuates between extremes of elation and despair and it's sometimes known as **bipolar depression** (as opposed to the more usual unipolar depression) because it hits both ends of the mood spectrum. An excellent personal account of this, which will also give you insight into the more regular forms of depression and the ways these relate to anger, is provided by David Wigoder in *Images of Destruction*.

SUICIDE

We cannot ignore that a small number of people who are depressed do kill themselves. A far, far greater number attempt to do so, or make some gesture towards it. Generally, more men than women actually complete the act, while more women than men attempt suicide. These proportions change, however, for different groups within society: so women doctors, for example, kill themselves just as often as their male counterparts, and three to four times more than other women.

Given the characteristics of depression that we talked about above – the intense sadness, loneliness and pain, the hopelessless that it will ever change, and the feeling that you're so useless or bad that everyone would be better off without you – it's clear that suicide is always a possibility in depression, though few people go so far as to make real plans. To think that killing yourself is an option can, on the one hand, provide almost a sense of relief (and in fact the majority of people do at some point in their lives contemplate the possibility); on the other hand, to consider it with any seriousness can be terrifying because of its extreme nature as a solution, especially if the methods considered are violent.

It is a great help to people to be able to actually admit that they've been thinking along these lines, but it's very difficult for friends and relatives not to show how appalled and even angry they are that such an apparently selfish action is being contemplated. Trying to talk someone out of their thoughts can be a dismal task. I remember years ago, before I considered psychology as a career, spending night after night 'talking reason' to my friend who continued to present me with quite logical arguments about why suicide was his only option. He was extremely intelligent and, apart from the fact that I deterred him by my presence, by the end of the night his determination was unshaken and I was wondering why on earth I chose to stay alive! There is no doubt that, if you are feeling suicidal, talking to people will help, but friends and relatives have too much to lose by your death, and you may feel you simply cannot tell them how desperate you actually are, so they are often less useful than a stranger. In a situation like this, it's usually better to make contact with the Samaritans or a good professional.

In his autobiography, *The Door Wherein I Went*, Lord Hailsham, whose brother had killed himself many years before, declares that 'Suicide is wrong, wrong, wrong.' There is no doubt that if someone close to you attempts suicide, it is a perfectly natural first reaction to feel very angry: it comes from feeling that you and your help and love have been rejected, and the person has been intensely selfish and not cared about you at all. It will be blended with guilt that you have somehow failed, and fear that next time he or she will succeed. If the attempt has been successful, these feelings will still be there, probably much more intensely, but the anger is often covered up with grief and guilt. Try to express it in any way you can because otherwise this mass of emotions will stay with you.

In his book, *Suicide and Attempted Suicide*, Erwin Stengel wrote: 'Most people who commit suicidal acts do not either want to die or to live; they want to do both at the same time, usually the one more, or much more, than the other.' If people really want to kill themselves, and get no help to deter them, then they rarely fail in the attempt. If their attempt is obviously serious then, without help, they will try again, whatever they say to the contrary. It is worth rescuing and being rescued; however angry a suicidal person may be at being hauled back from death, there is no doubt that time very often heals, especially if it contains experienced help. Al Alvarez, the poet and writer, describes in his book, *The Savage God*, how at one stage of his life, he was determined to die and made a very serious attempt to achieve this single-minded goal. Remarkably he failed, surviving long enough to find new meaning and happiness within his life.

Attempts which fail and which are not violent, such as taking non-lethal overdoses or cutting wrists and arms in a non-fatal manner, are usually the acts of much younger men and women, often adolescent, and should be taken seriously as a desperate 'cry for help'. In Stengel's words they are acts of people who may want to die (though this is not always the case), but who want more strongly to live. But however much these so-called para-suicides may actually prefer life, there is always a number who do actually die, often because they have failed to take into account the amount of alcohol they've consumed before overdosing, or because they have taken tablets, such as paracetamol, which are non-lethal in very small doses, but very dangerous in slightly larger ones.

Over the last 10 years suicide in young people has increased by 24 per cent. The figures may actually be higher, especially in the under 16's where coroners may record accidental death out of compassion for parents. The fact that a young person is depressed can often be mistaken for the more predictable moodiness, secrecy and lethargy of normal adolescent development, especially as communication between parents and children often breaks down for a period during adolescence. Keeping those channels open and criticism to a minimum might let you stay more aware of their despair if it exists.

If you're a young person feeling that life looks hopeless, then do find someone to talk to about your feelings and your fears. You may well feel you can no longer discuss things with your parents – most of us have spent a period of our lives unable to do this – but the Samaritans, or a school counsellor, or Nightline at university, will all listen and help. However bad these feelings are they *will* pass. It's true that you can probably see the bad aspects of the world more clearly in some ways than the adults who have grown used to them, but the alternatives are not just to learn to pretend they don't exist *or* to kill yourself. There is the third option to realise that everything and everybody (including your parents and you and the world) have both good and bad aspects, and you can keep your new clear vision to tackle the things you hate as you and your capabilities grow.

Despite the fact that suicide and its attempt are no longer regarded as criminal acts, there still remains a stigma attached to the action. That it is often regarded as selfish and cowardly may make you or your relatives share a sense of shame and guilt that can stop you seeking help. Such acts may be hidden within families or dismissed as 'attention-seeking'. Often they *are* attention-seeking – which I take to mean the inappropriate cries of people needing to be listened to – and should be treated accordingly. They always mean that something is wrong.

WHAT CAUSES DEPRESSION?

Over the centuries there have been very many theories about what makes a person suffer from what was once called melancholia and now is called depression. From personality to the weather, from thought patterns to hormonal imbalance, from early loss to diet, and many more besides. Our urge to find a single cause reflects our human need to reduce complexity, to make things as simple and as understandable as possible. But human beings are phenomenally complex and different to each other, and the causes for their moods, both happy and wretched, are infinite. It's not comfortable, however, to contemplate so much uncertainty, and it's not useful if we want to learn from the experience of others how to change our moods for the better. So we can and do describe broad categories of cause and these in turn affect the way we deal with our problems. What's important to remember is that you are unique, and you will rarely perfectly fit this explanation or that one, or even that one plus another. But it's the explanations that are inadequate – not you.

Medical explanations

There is no doubt that, when people are feeling really depressed, they suffer a number of physical symptoms which may end up seeming almost to paralyse them. There is also the risk of death through suicide. Because of these factors, the medical model sees depression as an illness. At its simplest it proposes that it is caused by alterations in the brain's chemistry: that certain neurotransmitters (or chemical messengers) which deliver the impulses or messages from one cell to another within the brain have reduced or are unable to get through for some reason. There is no proof for this gained from actually studying the chemistry of the brain, but rather from the fact that antidepressant drugs, designed to restore these messengers to their normal levels of activity, do have a certain level of effectiveness.

However, this only suggests that the brain's chemistry is altered during depression; it doesn't prove that a change in its chemistry *caused* the depression, and the fact that people who simply take antidepressant drugs and do not change themselves or their environment in any way will often find themselves depressed again when they stop taking them, suggests that other aspects might be more important.

One of the most usual divisions that many psychiatrists make in depression is between so-called **reactive** depression – where there is a clear external cause, such as bereavement or unemployment – and **endogenous** depression which they see as an illness caused entirely by changes in the brain's chemistry. 'Reactive' implies you are reacting to an obvious event; 'endogenous' means that the cause is located within you. Others feel that this division is simply a reflection of our lack of knowledge: that depression *always* has an external, or non-chemical, cause of some kind or another but for some sufferers this cause is not obvious to us, and so we call it endogenous.

Similarly, there is no evidence that heredity plays any part in causing depression. Although it may seem as if it runs from parent to child, it's clear that living with a depressed parent is bound to have an effect on the children. You know what it's like just to go to the pub for an evening with someone who is feeling wretched: there's little chance that you'll leave as happy as you entered, even with the help of a mind-altering drug like alcohol! There is no doubt that a depressed parent can become an overwhelming responsibility for a child, especially as it's true that they can never deal with the parent's unhappiness successfully, as much as they hope to do so.

There are certain physical conditions – illnesses such as hepatitis and various viruses, as well as hormonal changes such as those that occur post-natally – which do appear to be associated with subsequent depression. These are discussed in Chapter 7 along with more controversial causes, such as the male menopause.

In conclusion, we know that there is a relationship between our mood and our brain chemistry: certain things have physical effects either directly on mood (such as drugs and alcohol), or perhaps indirectly via illness or hormonal changes. However, there is no clear evidence that changes in brain chemistry actually *cause* depression. Moreover, attributing depression to this, or to a genetic structure that might produce it, tends to let us off looking at the complexity of our lives – both psychological and social – and may take away our own power and responsibility for change.

Psychological explanations

There are a number of theories within psychology and psychoanalysis which have been proposed over the years to explain why people become depressed. There is good evidence that each of these theories has merit, but, since depression is so much easier to describe than to explain, no one theory is ever likely to fit every individual's history.

The psychoanalytic theories concern happenings in the first few years of life and especially the relationships we have with our parents or caretakers, or the loss of such a relationship. It is important to remember that there is no such thing as a perfect upbringing: Freud (and a number of other great thinkers) considered that we were all psychologically damaged to some extent and that madness of all kinds was on a continuum with normality. In the same light, Donald Winnicott, a British psychoanalyst, considered that the best anyone could hope for and provide was 'good enough mothering'.

One fundamental root of depression, as explained within psychoanalysis, is the feeling of loss which comes about usually as a result of grieving which has never been properly completed. We rarely give a child the chance to talk about or to express his or her angry and sad feelings over the loss of someone close, as we do with an adult, and so they will often grow up carrying these hidden within them until some new experience of loss reawakens them. So the woman in her menopause (see Chapter 7) may become simply sad because of present losses – of fertility, children, youth, and perhaps a parent or husband – but depressed if these spark off some old unresolved experience.

Frank was in his mid-thirties and had a year ago separated from his wife, Helen. He had taken the five-year-old son, and Helen had the daughter, and the children spent each weekend together at alternate houses. It all seemed so well worked out. But Frank had become more and more depressed over the year, and was drinking an amount which alarmed his new partner and eventually scared him.

I can't do anything any more. I can't work properly; can't make love; get angry all the time with my son, and I just don't know why. I'm usually drunk when my daughter's here, so although I'd like it to be perfect, I'm wrecking that as well.

Obviously there were reasons to be sad: he'd lost his wife and to some extent his daughter. He'd changed homes and jobs, so he was bound to feel under considerable strain from such a series of life events. But it all felt more than that. Gradually, almost as if it was irrelevant, he told me about the tragedy of his childhood: the annual family holiday to Devon, his parents, his sister and him; when he was six his having measles just before they were due to leave; his mother staying back to care for him for a week while the others went on ahead; the drive down to join them, and the crash that killed his mother but left him physically untouched.

So the beautifully modern sophisticated arrangement of separation that he and Helen had devised so carefully, had reawakened the awful pain and guilt and anger that he'd felt over his mother's death. Once again he had lost someone he loved, and had actually 'caused' (in his eyes) the loss to occur; once again he felt the guilt of this and also the guilt of putting his son in the same position as he'd been in – separated from his mother with a morose, drunk, grieving father.

By no means all reactivated grief is so clearly demonstrated: you may not have recently lost someone yourself, but be affected by other people's losses, which wake up your own early sadness. You may find yourself particularly sensitive to 'being let down' by people. This seems rather different to separation, perhaps, but when a parent dies or leaves the child for any length of time, the child is going to feel let down in some sense. In fact it is the anger and rage that this causes which is most often swallowed by children as being unacceptable and then turned against themselves. It's not that experiencing early separations will make us all depressed – we all know cases to show this clearly isn't so – it's where the child is not given the same chance to grieve (see Chapter 3, pp. 32–35) that we accept in adults, that later problems may arise.

In a survey of working-class women in Camberwell, London, Brown and Harris found that around a quarter of these were depressed. This is far higher than the proportion of middle-class people and can partly be explained by the poverty of their environment. However, it's also true that working-class people lose their parents while they're children more often than others, and their research suggested that losing a mother before the age of 11 was an important factor in making the women more vulnerable to the depressing effects of recent major life events.

In the same way that early loss can be reawakened by later adult experiences, so can rejected love. Linda, described at the beginning of this chapter, saw her depression beginning when she had failed to be made departmental manager at her firm. Her boss, whom she admired, had led her to believe that the post would be hers, but then had given it to someone whom Linda had no time for. Over the course of therapy, she revealed that the feelings of rejection and betrayal ('being tricked') had been a feature of her life. Two years earlier her husband from whom she'd been separated, had asked her to leave her job and join him in London, which she did. Within a week he said he'd changed his mind, and sent her packing, jobless and homeless. A dreadful enough experience for anyone, that's true, but finally we reached an even earlier event. The second of two daughters, her family life had been full of strife. When she was nine, her mother had decided to leave her husband with one of the children. Her father asked Linda if she would stay with him and, although upset at the thought of rejecting her mother in this way, she agreed. He then decided her older sister would be more use in caring for him, and she was sent away to join her mother – rejected and betrayed, as well as full of guilt towards her mother for her initial choice.

A third type of early experience linked to later depression often occurs in middle-class high achievers: the businessman who runs an ever-growing string of companies; the hospital administrator who turns a backward hospital into an efficient, highly-thought-of service. And suddenly becomes depressed. For them the phrase 'only loved for what you can achieve' holds enormous emotional truth. The middle classes in particular raise their children to achieve, and the feeling that love is dependent on this is often very deeply ingrained and carried on and on through adulthood, like the proverbial carrot dangling in front of them. At some point (for example, if a parent dies or begins to dement, or if they realise they've reached as far as they are able), the pointlessness of all they've done hits them and depression sets in.

'What have I actually achieved? Oh, yes; I know the hospital's fine now; I know its reputation's turned full circle. So what? What does it actually matter in the world. What use is any of it really?'

Although the pointlessness is initially attached to their jobs, what they are really feeling is the pointlessness of ever trying to get the love they need from that parent long ago. Getting them to admit that the task is no longer possible, letting them grieve for the simple unqualified love, and even for the childhood they never felt they had, is an essential part of therapy.

Psychological theories when compared to psychoanalytical or Freudian, are not so different as they sometimes make out. A psychological theory that concerns past experiences is the 'learned helplessness theory' of depression proposed by Martin Seligman, a professor of psychology in Pennsylvania. In some earlier experiments it had been noticed that dogs that were given unpredictable electric shocks in situations from which they could not escape, developed a behaviour similar to depressed humans: compared to other dogs, they failed in the second part of the experiment to learn a means of escape. They simply lay down and whined quietly and accepted the shock passively. If occasionally the animal did manage to escape, it seemed unable to use this learning, as if it didn't 'believe' that this escape route would work a second time. Seligman suggested that depressed people have similarly suffered a number of cruel, uncontrollable blows in their lives and have learned to believe that they have no control over any events in the future.

Certainly, this learned helplessness is a feature of many people who come for help with their depression, especially the women. Gill had been a temporary secretary but had failed to get work from her agency after having a bad panic attack one day in her office. She had become depressed very rapidly, staying in bed most of the day, and sitting brooding all evening in front of the television. Her husband had issued her an ultimatum that she had to seek help or he would leave. She sat in her chair and stared at the wall with her face turned almost right away from me.

'I get the impression that you don't think there's much point being here,' I said. 'No point at all,' she mumbled. 'But your

doctor said your husband had issued some sort of ultimatum?'
'It'll make no difference. He'll go anyway.'

Over the next few weeks we pieced together her childhood: a mother who had died when she was three; a father who had abused her sexually from the age of eight and then walked out when she was 12; a series of foster homes which meant separation from her younger brother; pregnant by her first boyfriend who promptly rejected her; the birth that stopped her taking 'A' levels, and so on. A young life filled her with 'shocks' which seemed unpredictable and uncontrollable. Now she was married to a man, less intelligent than she, who seemed to care but knew no way to show it. I knew how he felt: Gill made it pretty difficult for anyone to show her love or caring, partly because she clearly did not see herself worth caring for, partly because whenever she had dared to come close to anyone she had been terribly hurt as a result, but also because of a long line of painful blows which had gradually made her feel that nothing she did would have any lasting effect and she was helpless to change the pattern of her life.

In the late seventies the 'learned helplessness' theory was changed a little. We all know that there are people who apparently are able to endure a long list of painful life events and still not become depressed. There are certainly large differences in how much we can take of what life has to chuck at us. The theory was reformulated to take this into account. It now proposes that it's not just the aversive, uncontrollable events which need to occur but a person needs to see the causes of those events as being to do with their own characteristics (for example, 'It occurred because I'm unlovable') rather than external circumstances ('. . . because he's such a cruel person'); as effecting all areas of their lives, so they can see no area where things will be all right; and as lasting forever, so nothing can be done to change things. For example, if a woman's husband leaves her, and she sees the cause of this that she's always been unlovable, this is something that concerns *her*, will affect other situations and circumstances around her, and will go on causing her grief all her life. Thinking about a difficult life event in this way will have a fundamental effect upon her behaviour: for example, she will stop trying to make relationships, since she will expect finally to be hurt and rejected.

So the way you think about the happenings in your lives will have clear effects upon your mood and behaviour. Another

American, the psychiatrist Aaron Beck, came to similar conclusions based on years of observing and talking to depressed people. He concluded that they had 'negative automatic thoughts' – ones that seemed to come from nowhere and showed a negative view of the self ('I'm useless'), the world ('this country's on its last legs'), and the future ('mankind will always be evil').

He noticed too that depressed people make 'symbolic logical errors', such as always providing a negative cause for an event ('he didn't say good-morning because he thinks I can't do my job properly'); seeing everything in black or white terms; and overgeneralising, so that one set-back is seen as ruining everything. He sees these ways of thinking as coming from assumptions about ourselves and life in general which are built up when we are young, and which, if we are to become and remain non-depressed, need to be challenged.

As with the possible changes in the brain's chemical structure that may appear with depression, it is also true that these pessimistic thought patterns may be a symptom of depression rather than actually causing the disorder. There is some evidence, however, that people who are depressed must learn to change this way of thinking in order to stay well in the future.

Dorothy Rowe also considers that certain assumptions about life provide excellent building blocks for the prison of depression. From these assumptions (for example, 'No matter how good and nice I *appear* to be, I am really bad, evil, valueless, unacceptable to myself and other people') we build life rules such as 'I must please everybody all the time'; 'I must never offend anybody'; 'It is wrong to get angry', and so on.

There are also psychological explanations of depression which do not concern themselves with either early experience or our thoughts and rules. These behavioural theories see depression as a lack of rewards (or 'reinforcement') in our lives; for example a lack of a desired social life may be one cause of depression. Your depressed mood will then be 'rewarded' since, when you first become depressed others often rally round you more than they did before (as depression continues, the reverse is true, with people actually staying away). The theory does not bother to ask why a person may lack friends in the first place, but simply looks to ways that the behaviours which might encourage friends can be increased (for example, by teaching social skills) and those which might force them away are decreased.

This sounds very simple, but it is often the best way initially to look at the problem when someone is so deeply depressed that they are doing practically nothing. For example, Lily, in her late sixties, had been hospitalised for deep depression. She lay in bed each morning on the ward, listening to Radio 3 and refusing to move or to dress herself. The nurses were getting pretty fed up constantly having to tell her and, when she finally slowly put on her last item of clothing, around midday, they hardly spoke another word to her. Looked at behaviourally, Lily had no reward for getting up – she could listen to her favourite music longer in bed, no one thanked her when she did finally dress herself, and there was nothing to do when she went to the day-room.

We contemplated banning the radio until she'd risen (or, worse still, switching it to Radio 1), but we decided to try *giving* rewards instead of taking them away. When Lily woke, we told her that she could have the special privilege of taking her radio into the day-room, so long as it wasn't too loud, and also, as soon as she was dressed, the nurse would go down to the canteen with her to have a cup of tea. She dressed with increasing speed each day, especially as the nurses had promised that the time they saved in nagging at her would now be spent in having proper conversations with her. Once real talking began in her life again, we were able to find out properly about Lily and what might have caused her depression.

Social theories of depression

When we look at the lives of the working-class women in Camberwell that Brown and Harris studied, we are not too surprised that a quarter of them were depressed. No psychological, medical or genetic theory of depression can explain away the fact that living in high-rise blocks of flats with small children, being frightened to walk alone at night, having no money for pleasure, no sense of the future, often without a companion to talk to about it all, is depressing. Very depressing.

Similarly Michael Banks from the Social and Applied Psychology Unit in Sheffield has followed a large group of 15-year-olds over a few years, through leaving school and getting jobs, or becoming unemployed. He and his team have found that psychological symptoms of emotional distress, including depression, go up when these young people are unemployed, and drop away when they get jobs. Although it certainly won't protect us from depression completely, having a job and some money and living in an environment which allows a community to develop is undoubtedly one defence against such distress.

Unemployment is a life event and chances are, if you are subject to some of the other social forces described above, you will have suffered a number of major events. Research has shown these to be clearly linked to depression as well as other illnesses (see Chapter 3, p. 30). Another reason why these social factors are depressing, is that people caught within them have often had little control over their lives and so their depression can clearly be seen within the 'learned helplessness' model (p. 84). This is why discovering areas, however small, that give you a sense of control, can be an important force against the oppression of relentless bad fortune, as can beginning to appreciate that it is this external oppression, not something about yourself, that is to blame.

Women, who suffer from depression far more commonly than men, are also more subject to situations that are uncontrollable. Although there have been some changes over the past 20 years, even middle-class women usually go through some years of dependency if they are to have children, and are less able to take personal control over countless aspects of their lives, both large and small. This may be one of the reasons they are more likely to become depressed.

Clearly no one theory explains everything for everyone, but perhaps we can join them to make some sort of generalisation. Perhaps people with difficult and uncontrollable early experiences – sometimes dramatically awful, and sometimes much more subtly undermining – learn to think about themselves in negative ways which encourage depression and which may make later fulfilling relationships more difficult to achieve. They therefore have fewer rewards in their lives, and some later negative event, however small, may be magnified to an extent which allows depression to begin in earnest. Because they are already pessimistic about themselves and their abilities to change things, and because they have fewer trusting relationships, they may not talk over their problems or go for help. And so on. This cycle alone is sufficient to explain depression in most sufferers. On top of this, if it all takes place in a framework of poverty, people are far more likely to suffer major life events, will have far more uncontrollable daily hassles, and are less likely to be able to find rewarding experiences within their lives.

WHAT HELP IS AVAILABLE?

The type of help that is offered for depression, as in other psychological problems, depends upon whom you approach, since how that person views the cause of depression will affect the way he or she treats it. Thus general practitioners and psychiatrists are quite likely to try you on a course of antidepressant medication. Those who practise a psychoanalytically oriented psychotherapy will foresee a series of sessions to consider what lies behind your depression; a cognitive therapist will give you exercises to challenge and change the thought patterns that keep your depression going; and a behaviour therapist will help you to introduce new rewards into your life and to remove the aspects that make you feel worse.

If you go to your general practitioner for depression the course of action he or she decides upon will depend upon their confidence and experience and time in dealing with the problem themselves, and their confidence and knowledge of local psychiatric and psychological services. As was discussed in Chapter 2, research has suggested that other forces may determine the treatment chosen: men are more likely to be sent for specialist help than women; women are more likely to be given minor tranquillisers and antidepressants than men; the middle classes are more likely to be sent for psychotherapy than the working classes, as are those who are younger and those who are more attractive – and so on. While most of this research was done in the United States, there is no reason to believe that British doctors (or anyone else for that matter) should be any less subject to unconscious bias in their decision-making.

Drug treatment

One of the main arguments for depression involving a change in the brain's chemistry comes from the fact that antidepressant drugs do successfully improve mood in a substantial proportion of people. In a large trial in the US which is considering these drugs and psychotherapy, assessments at the end of the trial have shown substantial improvements in those on antidepressants in 60 per cent of patients, slightly higher than the therapy groups. However, other research shows that drug effects are not so long-lasting, while therapy may be expected to extend with time. There is no doubt therefore, that antidepressants may be useful taken as a short course in order to lift your mood sufficiently to change aspects of your life for the better. Leslie told about her experiences:

My marriage had ended about three months previously and I was gradually realising that I was pretty depressed. Nevertheless, I applied for a job in another town – almost as something to do. A week later I felt worse than ever and broke down in front of my doctor. She put me on a course of antidepressants and after a couple of weeks I started feeling much less hopeless. About the same time I had an interview for the job and was offered it. The move was really good for me and I've never looked back. I think the drugs helped me to think more positively again and to get the job. I don't think I'd have even made the interview without them.

Although the difference between a depressive illness (or endogenous depression), and a depressive reaction (where an unhappy event can be identified) is thought by many not to be particularly useful, doctors often use it as a rough guide to prescribing either antidepressants, or anxiolytics (tranquillisers) respectively, but in cases of doubt they will usually prescribe the former. So long as you don't think of drugs as a magic cure-all, and so long as you use them as a temporary crutch while you get on with sorting out your life, then they can certainly be useful. But do make sure you discuss their effects, both good and bad, with your GP, or psychiatrist, so that they know which particular brand and dosage is correct for you, and, if you find the depression returns when you stop the drugs, then do seek from them or from the recommendations of others, some form of psychotherapy to help you change the basis of your depression.

As was discussed in Chapter 2, there are two main groups of drugs prescribed for depression. The first, most generally effective and therefore most commonly used, are the tricyclics, and the others are the monoamine-oxidase inhibitors (MAOIs). You can tell which you are taking since the MAOIs require quite strict dietary control to prevent high blood pressure occurring; for example, you will be told not to eat cheese, broad beans, Bovril (or any form of yeast extract) or herrings. Nor should you take any other form of drug, not even cough syrup, without consulting your doctor. They take around three weeks for the effects to be notice-able. Their principal side-effect is dizziness, especially when you stand up, but you may also experience constipation, dry mouth, headache, tremor, agitation, rashes, and problems with urinating. There should be at least two weeks between taking a tricyclic antidepressant and one of the MAOI group.

The tricyclic group take up to two weeks to become active, and are effective in the short term in 60 to 70 per cent of patients. They usually bring swift relief to sleep problems and restore appetite. Some have a relaxing effect for those who are also suffering anxiety, while others are less tranquillising. Side-effects may begin at once; as usual, they vary with individuals and with different drugs, and your doctor needs to be kept informed. Generally speaking, this group of drugs may produce drowsiness, reduced sex drive, urinary retention, nausea, sweating, dry mouth, tremor, or constipation.

Lithium, usually prescribed as a preventive drug in manic depression, is sometimes given in depression alone where other drugs have failed. It's discussed in detail in Chapter 14. Preferably no drugs should be taken long term, and their usefulness should be regularly reviewed by the doctor.

For anyone who is so severely depressed that they have become almost completely inactive, there can be a real risk of suicide once antidepressants have begun to work – simply because they are pulled into a more motivated frame of mind. People in this situation need particular care until their mood lifts *past* the sui-cidal stage.

Hospitalisation and ECT

Largely speaking, people are hospitalised for depression if they are so depressed, agitated or withdrawn that they are not caring for themselves physically, or if there is a risk of suicide. If you are actually making attempts to kill yourself, you may be legally forced, or 'sectioned', to go into hospital as a protection to yourself (see Chapter 2, pp. 19–20). Of course, few people welcome the prospect of hospital, but at its best, it provides peace and understanding and a sanctuary from the stresses that provoke depression. At its worst, people describe their feelings of shame at being in such a place; they are surprised in some hospitals, at how little of the 'talking' therapies are provided, and that the majority of treatments involve drugs or ECT (shock treatment). However, over the past few years psychiatric nursing training has improved enormously, and so some form of additional therapy is usually combined with physical treatments.

ECT is used more for depression than for any other disorder (see Chapter 2, pp. 18–19). Many people are surprised, when first they are in-patients, at the frequency with which ECT is still used in many hospitals. In about two-thirds of people with severe depression it has a swift effect upon symptoms, but this is not necessarily long-lasting, and controversy remains concerning the seriousness of its subsequent memory loss. Nevertheless, if drugs have not proved themselves useful in someone in deep depression, ECT may bring their mood and activity to a level where they can take part in therapy. Except in the most severe of cases, a consent form is usually required for ECT.

Experiences of hospitalisation vary enormously, both because of differences between hospitals and between wards, but also because what you need of a hospital will vary for different individuals. George described his experience:

> *At best I'd felt like running away for ever; at worst, of course, I could see no way other than topping myself. Hospital let me get my head together and start to think clearly about my life. Where it had been and where I'd like to go. I knew that when I went out it was all going to be facing me again, but it was the first chance I had to breathe – to actually get my head above water and see what was happening. That was so helpful because I got a quite different perspective out of it that's lasted over the nine months since I came out. A good guest-house might have done the same, but I wouldn't have gone there, that's the difference!*

A hospital also should provide a place to share your experiences and your feelings, to help others and to gain new skills and approaches to life outside. The availability of resources within hospitals also varies enormously, and, if you or someone close to you is likely to be admitted, the more research you can do on the choices available to you, the better your experience will be.

Psychological therapies

The therapy that a psychologist or psychotherapist will offer you will depend upon their ideas about the causes of depression. Some of the methods are discussed or implied in the section on causation, but it is worth following through the case of Linda to show the different ways that it could be approached.

First, the issue of trust had to be dealt with. If anyone had been let down as often as Linda, then difficulty in trusting people would be an issue with everyone, including the therapist. Chances are Linda would look for the slightest hint of criticism to decide that I did not really like her, but was just seeing her because it was my job to do so. She would take quite a long time to accept that she could be cared for for herself, and she would find this very uncomfortable for some time because it would put her at risk of being tricked and rejected. At the end of one session, I told her that I was going to be unable to see her the following week, for a good cause, and would therefore fit her in on the Saturday morning. She turned up very tight-lipped and cold, and I suggested that she seemed angry with me.

'Well, I am as a matter of fact,' she stated. 'You obviously think I'm a real looney if you don't think I can go a week without seeing you. I thought you had a bit of confidence in me, but I can see now that you don't.'

That put me in my place, but it also allowed us to consider her negative interpretation of what had happened: she preferred to see me as thinking poorly of her than to accept that I cared enough to give up part of my weekend.

She needed to deal with the losses in her life. She had never grieved for the break-up of her marriage, and still half believed that her husband would arrive again to sweep her off her feet. Eventually she learned to let herself cry in front of me (without trying to laugh at the same time in case I thought her weak or stupid), and then to accept the sadness that her marriage had really ended. This allowed her to begin building something more satisfying with her present boyfriend.

She needed to really let out some of the rage that she felt about those who had let her down so badly: her boss for a start, but also her husband and, most importantly, her father. Once she could accept how much she hated him for his betrayal, once she could admit that she'd wanted him dead, she could then begin to realise that you can both love and be angry with the same person. That admitting how bad she found his behaviour didn't destroy her love for him, but rather let her feel more. It is widely appreciated that depression occurs when anger that should have been directed towards another is turned in on yourself. This happens because a child can rarely accept that a parent has done something very wrong. Only when this anger is finally acknowledged and expressed outwards can you start to like yourself once more.

All this could be explored in a psychodynamic way; that is, by using the relationship with me, as her therapist, to experience the way she dealt with others, both now and in the past. When these feelings had surfaced and she had gained insight into their origins, we moved into a more cognitive-behavioural mode and I began to teach her to challenge some of her negative thoughts about the current events in her life. She still felt bad about not getting the job she'd hoped for, and by keeping a diary of feelings and the thoughts that precipitated them, we found she was still thinking that her boss thought her inferior in some way. I learnt that she had never asked him for feedback on her interview or on her performance generally. We went over the 'worst scenario': what was the worst possible thing he could say to her if she asked him? She decided it would be to be told she was completely incompetent and would be moved to a less senior position. This was extremely unlikely but even if it occurred, it was no worse than her fantasies about his opinion, so she agreed she might as well ask. When they finally talked it turned out he had been very embarrassed about the whole promotion. He had wanted her for the job but had been leaned upon by a senior colleague to promote a family friend. Her relief was spectacular and the lesson she learnt was not to mind-read – humans have never shown that it's possible!

She spread this knowledge into her home relationship as well and, since she and her boyfriend had slipped into a boring routine which each blamed on the other, they also agreed to go out together twice a week, and make love at least twice a week. To practise expressing her feelings she agreed to make one 'I resent you for . . .' statement each day, and one 'I appreciate you for . . .' statement. It may sound mechanistic, but people sometimes need to be forced back into good habits – even those of appreciating each other and enjoying themselves! And it worked wonders for their relationship.

This is a case where a wide range of psychological therapies were applied. Because research shows that one therapy has little advantage over another on the whole, and I believe in the usefulness of each, used appropriately, I take an eclectic, or wide-ranging, approach. However, an expert in any one form of therapy is likely to have equally good results, especially as researchers are beginning to emphasise that differences between therapists clearly contribute to the difference between success and failure.

There are no psychotherapies designed in themselves to change governments, increase jobs or improve town-planning. However, by dealing with your depression in any of the ways above you will feel more powerful, more in control of your own destiny, and more able to take on councils and social services and errant spouses. This will be much easier if you are part of a group, whether it's specifically for depression or more generally for helping with parenthood, unemployment, or simply a local tenants' association. In a recent study of people who cope very well with unemployment, many of them were found to be politically active in some way, or else involved in voluntary organisations. They worked longer hours than they had ever done for money, they were broke, but they were certainly not depressed.

Self-help

You can follow some of the psychological strategies for yourself. You can introduce areas of reward into your life; you can turn large-scale plans that seem impossible into small steps that are achievable and provide satisfaction; you can, to some extent, challenge negative thoughts that bring you down. But because of your depression and feelings of pointlessness you may also wonder, why bother?

Why bother sounds much more rational if you are alone with your depression and your experiences. Perhaps, therefore, one of the most useful strategies of self-help is to join or form some sort of group. Social support – which means having someone in whom you can confide and who confides in you – has been shown again and again to be an important protection against depression, even for those people who have suffered many of the life events that might be thought to cause it. At least, try to find one person with whom you can have this type of relationship; alternatively take part in some group activity which allows discussion of these issues.

Admitting that you are depressed to others may be the way to admitting it to yourself: it may make your feelings and actions more understandable, and so increase the possibility of change. Hearing that others feel the same way can lessen your feelings of isolation, and realising that others share your experiences can also lead to greater understanding of the forces that make us what we are. The women's movement has been particularly valuable in this field in terms of consciousness-raising groups and group work in women's therapy centres. Moreover, most voluntary organis-ations such as befriending services like Homestart and Newpin, provide help primarily aimed at women. There is nothing unfair in this: it is women who suffer most depression and women with young children who are most isolated. At the same time, there are very large numbers of men who are depressed too, but who may mask their depression in alcohol or work. Men's upbringings make it more difficult for them to open up to each other, and because of this they often deny themselves a vital form of comfort. Bringing up our children, whether they're boys or girls, in a way that makes it permissible for them to cry and to get angry, as well as to be joyful for themselves, will help rule out some of the inequalities as adults.

Going into and coming out of a depression can involve a long and difficult path; that's indisputable. But once you've travelled it – confronted painful feelings, shared sadness and discovered new pleasures – things rarely seem so bad again. Once you know you've been down in the pit, survived and come out again, chances are you'll find in yourself a new strength with which to confront the future.

Chapter

Mind and body: physical aspects of psychological problems

In the eighteenth century Descartes, the French philosopher, proposed that mind and body were separate parts of nature: that the human body was a machine with 'a ghost' in it which was the mind. This century in particular has seen many arguments against this division, as we've learnt more and more about how intimately connected the two aspects of the person really are. More recent arguments see different parts of the mind affecting each other just as much as they affect different parts of the body, and vice versa. You experience your body both through your eyes and ears and touch, and through your mind in terms of how you feel you are, what shape you are, how you want to be, and so on.

This development comes alongside the growth of knowledge which has let us see how frequently physical illnesses are related to stress of some sort, and how some physical illnesses seem to cause psychological problems. We are still far from understanding how these psychosomatic problems come about, but at least we can now realise that both mind *and* body need looking after, whether the problem is regarded as physical or mental.

PHYSICAL ILLNESSES AND PSYCHOLOGICAL PROBLEMS

There are physical illnesses, some of whose symptoms mimic those of psychological problems. For example, hyperthyroidism (an over-active thyroid gland) is sometimes mis-diagnosed as anxiety (see Chapter 4) since restlessness, poor sleep and concentration, and feelings of apprehension and tension are almost always found in the illness. One of the signs that distinguishes the two conditions is that, if you are suffering from hyperthyroidism, you will find heat difficult to tolerate and your appetite will increase despite the fact that you are losing weight. Hypoglycaemia (low blood sugar) can provide a variety of symptoms which resemble depression and anxiety, and depression is often seen in illnesses such as hepatitis and glandular fever.

Recently it has been realised that there are a number of conditions linked to viruses, about which little is known but which often have depression and anxiety, alongside dreadful muscle tiredness, as part of the symptom pattern. These viruses may take months or even years to recover from and, due to the lack of knowledge about them yet, you may be treated as though your symptoms are psychological only, and so sent for psychiatric help. One such illness now has the grand name of myalgic encephalomyelitis, for which there is a support group listed at the end of the book.

When you are delirious, you will often see and hear frightening things and may hold quite paranoid fears about the people around you. You may also be confused about your surroundings and about time. Delirium is usually caused by high temperature, especially in children, but can also be a side-effect of drugs, or an inappropriate mix of them, or as part of withdrawal effects from drugs or alcohol. Although it might appear that delirious people are behaving or talking in a very mad manner, it almost always vanishes with treatment of the underlying condition.

There are of course many physical illnesses that result in depression simply because they affect your life in some negative way; for example, the chronic and disabling pain of arthritis; or the knowledge that you are HIV positive and so an AIDS carrier; the diagnosis of a life-threatening disease such as cancer, and so on. None of these necessarily produces depression, but the likelihood is obviously increased by their presence. Peter Maguire's research in Manchester on women after mastectomy gave the sad news that almost half were suffering from depression. However, this is quite likely to be the result of a lack of communication during the build-up to the operation, and is clearly not an inevitable result. An encouraging on-going study by Mary Burton which is taking place in Coventry, suggests that if a brief personal talk with a surgeon about the operation and the woman's feelings, takes place before surgery, subsequent depression is reduced considerably. Although such conversations are going to be an unusual occurrence for some time, the same result is likely to be achieved by talking to anyone you feel will understand or will hold information that you need, or by finding out (for example, from the Samaritans or your local information office) if there is a cancer support group in your area. The addresses for the mastectomy and colostomy societies are given at the end of the book. AIDS counselling services are being set up swiftly in each city, and again established agencies will provide local addresses.

There are a number of drugs which can have depression as a side-effect; for example, antibiotics and the contraceptive pill. If you find yourself becoming depressed for apparently no reason, and you've recently begun a course of medication for some physical problem, it is worth checking out the side-effects with your doctor. There is often an alternative which may be better for you.

It has been strongly suggested for some years that diet may be linked to conditions such as hyperactivity in children (though the results of research have been disappointing), and migraine. More recently, alongside the general interest and acceptance of the importance of a good diet, a number of health workers have begun to suggest that even severe mental problems may have a dietary basis. In his book, *Not All in the Mind*, Dr Mackarness suggests that some people may have an intolerance or allergy to certain foods (and especially to those they like most) which, unlike the rashes or sickness produced in other allergies, may create mental symptoms rather than physical ones. Although much of this work is still speculative, there seems little to lose by those suffering distressing psychological problems in testing out guesses about diet.

On the other side of the coin are all the illnesses that appear to be related to experiencing stress. This does not mean that stress alone will be sufficient to produce a physical illness, but that it is one of the factors which might make you susceptible. As was pointed out in Chapter 3, the range of illnesses is enormous: diabetes, cold, cancer, heart disease, influenza, asthma, eczema and other skin complaints, rheumatoid arthritis, lower back pain, and so on. It may be that *any* illness for which we have a susceptibility, through heredity, or through exposure to viruses or any environmental hazards (smoking, asbestos, radiation, pollution, or whatever), has more chance to take effect if we experience particular stress. What this means is that all physical illnesses may be psychosomatic (have a psychological factor involved in the cause), and so should be treated both physically and psychologically to some extent.

Seeing a psychiatrist or psychologist may well help to relieve some of the frustration you feel about your condition, and allow you to live with it while it lasts more easily, and this may speed up the cure which still comes mainly from the passage of time, rest, and possibly from improved diet.

Because the links between mind and body are so active, it may be that we can never clearly decide whether the illness causes the mood change, or vice versa. This is shown by the fact that, even with the illnesses mentioned above, it has been noticed that patients were often stressed or mildly unhappy when their physical problems began. So another explanation might be that their stress made them more susceptible to infection (which happens because the auto-immune system, which normally fights off such infections, becomes less efficient during stress), and the illness itself makes them feel helpless, a state that's often linked to depression (Chapter 6, p. 84).

HYPOCHONDRIA

Hypochondria, or hypochondriasis as it's called in psychiatric classifications, is the name given to the disorder in which you are worrying constantly about your health: worrying that is completely out of proportion to any evidence that exists for any disease. Since it's occasionally used in a critical way, behaviour therapists have suggested it should be called 'illness phobia', or simply anxiety. If you are suffering from an anxiety state (Chapter 4), many of you will become concerned over a particular aspect of your health, mainly because the symptoms of anxiety are often physical, and so it's natural to wonder if your palpitations or your bowel movements or your headaches, and so on, are normal. It's always important to have yourself checked over physically. The problem comes when you still cannot get the possibility out of your mind: when there is always a second, third, fourth . . . opinion to be sought, or when you spend a long time and possible pain and discomfort having more and more tests and even unnecessary operations.

Worrying constantly over health is also a feature of obsessional-compulsive disorders (see Chapter 8), depression (Chapter 6), agoraphobia (Chapter 5), as well as anxiety. Whatever the over-riding problem, the difficulty you are faced with is that, whatever tests, operations and specialists you try, you will *never* be satisfied or reassured – there will always be something else that could be done – and so you need to find and tackle the root of the problem.

Shirley was a librarian and the head of her department. She came for help because she was clearly very depressed, but during the interview she raised several times that she'd been suffering pain in her abdomen which her doctor had diagnosed as a spastic colon. She had had numerous unpleasant tests and examinations – all negative – and was now being treated with antidepressants. She mentioned that she also had a bad back and that her left arm kept aching, but that the doctor thought it was nothing. Her husband had been made redundant two years earlier, and she wondered if she should take early retirement because she felt so unwell all the time, and so that she could keep him company. Her mother had died recently; although she used to live with Shirley, her husband had found it too much to have her there and so she'd spent her last two years in a home.

There's no classic picture of hypochondria – most of us have little twinges of it, but real sufferers have a variety of symptoms and backgrounds. However, Shirley illustrates some common points. First, her husband (and wives can do this just as well) had an interest in keeping her feeling poorly; he really did want her at home with him. This became obvious because, as she began to lose her symptoms, he began to get upset and ask what his role would be if she could do everything for herself. In other men and women, the partner will only give support and affection when they are ill, so their pains and symptoms are rewarded. Second, she was very angry with her husband, although it was previously unacknow-ledged, because she felt he'd forced her to put her mother in a home. Pent-up anger is very often linked to physical disease, especially arthritis and back pain. Third, reassurance by me, by her doctor, her specialist or anyone else she asked didn't work at all in the long term; in fact, it had to be stopped since at some stage

Shirley had to live with and learn to control her anxiety without reassurance. Finally, it turned out that they'd stopped making love two years earlier when her husband had had some angina. A poor or absent sex life is again quite common in people with problems of hypochondria.

After some initial individual sessions, her husband was brought in too, and his worries about a lack of role and about the possible risks to his health that sex would entail were talked about openly at last. Both of them were taught to express their needs and their appreciations of and resentments against the other; that is, they were taught to talk to each other about their feelings, both positive and negative. Shirley was taught relaxation and various cognitive strategies to help stop her worrying, and her husband was forbidden to reassure her. Finally, they were given some strategies to help their love-making begin again without anxiety.

Often it's necessary to look at some underlying fear or guilt or anger. One young man, newly married, came to see his doctor again a few months after he had successfully had a cyst removed. Now he was depressed and looked dreadful, and was describing pain in his chest and a constant cough. The doctor talked to him about what had been happening to him in the last few years: that his mother had died with breast cancer and his grandfather with throat cancer, only weeks before the wedding. He'd not let the event be postponed because he felt that was wrong, and he'd not cried properly because that was 'unmanly'. Pointing out the links between his pains and those of his mother and grandfather, and letting him know it was OK to cry and to grieve, was simple but remarkably effective.

No one denies your pain in hypochondria. The body is quite capable of producing quite agonising pain to reflect some of the conflicts or emotions you can't express in other ways. But, if you find yourself constantly doubting the results of tests or opinions, then it will pay your peace of mind to begin to consider the psychological causes that may lie behind the physical pain.

IS IT THE HORMONES?

Hormones certainly can produce psychological problems if there's too much or too little of them: we've mentioned that above in discussing hyperthyroidism. They are also quite likely to be part of the cause of some adolescents' problems, of premenstrual tension (PMT) and postnatal depression, and the low mood experienced by some women taking the contraceptive pill. Women certainly suffer more depression than men, and it might be thought that their more frequent periods of hormonal change could be a cause of this. However, the research on sex differences more and more suggests that the differences in depression rates are as likely to be the result of different life experiences as of anything biological.

Premenstrual tension

Premenstrual tension has been discussed in the medical literature for the past 50 years. Just how many women suffer from it is not clear since the proportion found (from 36 per cent to 95 per cent) has varied with how widely the problem is defined. Nevertheless, it's clear that a lot of women do experience any or all of the following: swollen breasts, headache, backache, cramps, tension, irritability, depression, feelings of loneliness, forgetfulness, swift mood changes, tiredness, sleep loss, unusual dreams, and many more.

Some writers, such as Katerina Dalton, argue that PMT is caused by a relative lack of the hormone progesterone during the build-up to a period, and she reports good results if this is supplemented by the use of progesterone suppositories or daily injections. Many women dislike these methods, however, and there is now an increasing number of synthetic progestogens on the market, which you can take in tablet form and which are reported to be quite effective in reducing some of the worst of the problems. You should discuss this with your doctor to see what he or she advises.

Although physical reasons clearly have a place in the overall explanation for PMT, they're not enough on their own. For example, many women who suffer from PMT do not do so before every period; rather, it happens when other difficulties are occurring in their lives. For example, Sandra described it like this:

Last month I felt particularly wretched just before my period. I screamed at my sons for not clearing up their crumbs after themselves each time they made a sandwich. They're almost in their twenties; it didn't seem much to ask. Everything looked so futile, so pointless. Keep going to work, coming home, cleaning up the mess, cooking the meals, cleaning more mess, and so on: round and round in ever-decreasing circles! With my period, it's as if the monthly cycle sometimes really emphasises the non-stop cycle in the rest of my life. As if sometimes the hormonal change in my body nudges me and says, 'Here you are again. Another month gone and everything just the same as ever.'

In the same way people describe becoming depressed in autumn or in spring. While some explanations for the autumn concern changes in the levels of sunlight as the days become shorter, Alvarez, in his book *The Savage God*, describes the effects of the spring cycle as follows: 'The impulse to take one's life increases in the spring not because of any mysterious biological change but because of the lack of it. Instead of change, there is stasis.' This process may well be a psychological factor present in PMT.

In recent years a change of emphasis away from the hormonal explanation alone suggests that actually learning to expect physical and psychological changes in yourself pre-menstrually makes the changes less severe, probably because it puts *you* more in control of them. The other clear message is to avoid stress as much as possible during that time. Keeping a diary to rate the level of your various symptoms, and recording what was happening in your life before each period will give you an idea of what to avoid or increase during that time.

Finally, a third cause and treatment is advocated in a new book, *Beat PMT Through Diet*. Maryon Stewart, the author, argues that PMT is more common nowadays because our diet has become so bad. She advises cutting down on coffee and sugar and salt, in particular; eating plenty of greens and limiting dairy products. Other writers have recommended vitamin B_6, and, more recently, preparations containing oil of evening primrose have been reported as bringing some relief.

This seems an easy and sensible way to start tackling your problems, though keeping a diary in addition will give you a better idea of what works best and of other aspects that might be affecting you. Your sense of control will certainly be raised by tackling the problem yourself.

The menopause

The depressed mood that some women suffer during the menopause is also only partially explained by hormonal changes. There are ways in statistics that you can estimate the role played in causation by different factors, and when you enter the fact that many women around that age have had a run of life events there remains no significant part to be played by hormones! They have, for example, seen their children leave home, their youth end, their parents (often) die, their husband perhaps lose interest. What you are looking at is loss – of children, of youth, of parents, of your reproductive selves – and no new ways yet learnt to feel productive and useful once again. Many of the points made on grieving in Chapter 3, will apply and be helpful during this period.

The *male* menopause is often talked about in the media. The picture we're usually given is of a man in his forties or fifties who's suddenly given up his wife and children (if they're still at home) to live with a much younger woman. He will often change his dress to look more fashionable, and may behave in many ways similar to his own sons. This behaviour seems so sudden and so out of character that it's not surprising that it appears to be only explained by a change in his body's chemistry.

There is no such thing as a male menopause. What these men are suffering from, in much the same way as the women, is a developmental crisis as they look back at their lives and on towards the sudden realisation of the inevitability of death. Norman described it like this:

I was 42 and I'd been married for 18 years. The boys were adolescent and giving us both a pretty awful time. I suspected I'd gone as far in the firm as I was going, and I felt pretty resentful about that. I used to dream about sitting behind the MD's desk and now realistically I knew this was highly unlikely. I could watch young people shooting up the ladder behind me. Looking back, I guess I'd been feeling pretty depressed for a couple of years. I didn't say anything to Mary. We'd been in such a rut for ages, and not talking about ourselves was part of it: the boys were taking up all our energies, and I suppose I resented that a lot too. When I looked at the future, it was ghastly: I realised it was going on and on like this. No prizes. No miracles. This was it for the other half of my life.

> *Then I was given a new secretary. She was young and bouncy and full of life and when I was with her she made me feel like I mattered again to someone. Not surprisingly, I made sure I was with her more and more. It seemed like everything would be OK if I could start all over again with her. I left Mary within a couple of months, and went to live in Ali's little flat. Really, it was awful. Half the time I could pretend to be a gay young blade with an exciting future, and the other half I felt like an octogenarian already, just comparing myself to her and her friends. The inevitable happened: Ali went off with someone else, and I tried to creep back to Mary, but she didn't want me. I made a suicide attempt – a reasonably serious one – and was sent to a psychiatrist. It's been a help, and I've understood a lot more about this time of life and how it often involves the end of dreams. I know my behaviour was an attempt to keep them going and to not look at the ordinariness of life and learn to accept it. But I'm still pretty lonely.*

Often both men and women act less dramatically but just as destructively by beginning to drink heavily. Both are ways to avoid facing the sadness – common but completely natural – that comes with the end of dreams of how it 'ought' to be. Only when this sadness is experienced and come to terms with can you begin to move on positively once again.

Postnatal depression

A time when huge hormonal changes and life changes take place together is following the birth of a child:

> *After we have given birth it is as if we wake up to discover that a mountain of sand has been deposited in front of the doors of our home. Some women get to work, energetically to dig routes out. They have friends who come along and help. They work round the sand and over the sand; they find marvellously inventive ways to cope with the situation. Some women find one difficult route out and stick to that. Some try to dig a way through and get buried, others just look at it, feel defeated, retreat within their four walls and give up.*

This is Vivienne Welburn's description of the post-birth period from her excellent book *Postnatal Depression* in which she talks about her own experiences and those of others. Like other depressions, these may have physical causes or psychological ones or both. As Welburn points out, however, considering 'the most common complication of the period following childbirth' solely as physical or psychological ignores the possible *social* causes – 'the essential question of why the sand need be there in the first place'.

Around half of all women suffer 'the blues' in the first few days after birth. They find themselves tearful, with problems of sleeping; they feel sad and irritable. For most of them the feelings end within a week, but for around 10 to 15 per cent they continue for a couple of months and around half of these will still be suffering from depression a year later. During postnatal depression women suffer from tiredness, anxiety, irritability, low spirits, a lack of sexual desire, guilt, and worry about their health. Despite the fact that hospital booklets on having a baby describe the possibility of these problems, many women still go on without help, thinking that it is all part of the changes that are bound to occur when you become a mother.

One or two women in every thousand suffer a much more severe form of mood disturbance generally referred to as post-puerperal psychosis. Within the first two weeks of birth they become agitated, can't sleep, and may have hallucinations (seeing or hearing things that aren't there) or delusions (believing things that aren't real), often about the baby. They may be obsessional, checking and re-checking things, paranoid that someone will harm them or their baby, or more clearly deeply depressed. They will usually be hospitalised for a couple of weeks, often with the baby, and treated with major tranquillisers or ECT. However, in Nottingham, some mothers are now being successfully treated out of hospital using community services and Homestart, the voluntary befriending agency.

It remains a matter of debate whether the blues, postnatal depression and puerperal psychosis are all different degrees of the same problem, and whether they are caused by changes in brain chemistry (and so treated with drugs or ECT), or by hormonal change, or by psychological or social factors – or any combination of these. In her book, *Depression After Childbirth*, Katerina Dalton argues that the massive hormonal changes that occur at birth can clearly account for the majority of cases seen. Certainly other hormones, such as those released by the thyroid gland, have well-verified effects upon mood, so there is no reason to doubt that changes in progesterone, in particular, may equally be concerned with depression, and she describes good results obtained by hormone injections or suppositories. Hormone treatment is still not common in Britain but it is worth discussing it with your general practitioner, particularly if you have found other drug treatments to be unsuccessful.

Although it is likely that a physical element *is* present in many postnatal depressions, nevertheless there are women who suffer from both the depressive and the psychotic form who have not given birth, but adopted a baby. Clearly there are other causes at work as well. These may be psychological in terms of early experience; for example, the woman who was brought up to feel responsible for her mother's happiness and who, inevitably, failed to provide it, may feel overwhelmed by the sudden responsibility of providing all aspects of happiness to her child. From a cognitive point of view, a woman who blames herself for what goes wrong and who has negative thoughts about her abilities is likely to get particularly upset and guilty at the inevitable constant minor hassles with her baby: the crying problems, the nappy rash, sleep and eating difficulties and so on. From a behavioural stance, such a massive life change means that old rewards may well no longer exist and new ones need to be created.

Of course, socially we provide plenty of causes for postnatal depression. Motherhood is completely unrewarded in our society; the media present a rosy view of perfect children who are always well-provided for, far from the reality of most; few women manage to maintain both babies and their career and so lose a valuable source of self-esteem; those that do suffer conflict and guilt about doing neither role correctly. And so on. Women tend to blame themselves and, to a lesser extent, their babies for what has happened to them. Looking at society's causes is not so easy to do when you are isolated and lonely, but using a women's group or a voluntary agency such as Homestart or Newpin, will let you realise that the pressures upon you are real and are shared by millions, and this alone can bring enormous relief. Newpin was started in London in response to the high levels of child abuse, family distress and maternal depression, and uses volunteer mothers to befriend others. The following quotes come from a recent article on its success: 'Newpin helped me clean out the cupboard of all the nasty things that had happened to me – I feel better and could put it all behind me'; 'I got what I expected from Newpin and more. The more is to be tolerant, to come to respect others' views and to know it is okay to cry'; 'I was isolated, I didn't know anyone on the estate; my mother and father died when I was five. They were like family to me at Newpin.' The support that such voluntary agencies can provide is obviously enormous.

So, just like all the other types of psychological problems, whether hormones may be involved or not, postnatal depression shows the usual complexity of causes: diet, aspects of the environment and society, psychological conflicts which are present at various developmental stages in your life, from childhood to old age, all have a part to play. Just as there is no one simple cause for these disorders, neither is there one single method to put things right. We should in fact be pleased about this: we are not automatons to be all lumped together, presumed to respond to the same things in the same way and to be treated all alike.

The way our minds and bodies work together is enormously complex, and we are never likely to understand it fully. The important thing is to tackle the physical, psychological and social factors that are apparent to some extent in all disease and all dis-ease.

Chapter

8

Obsessive-compulsive disorders

Every time I touch wood or throw salt over my shoulder I am responding in a minute way to an obsessional thought: something dreadful will happen if I don't do this. The thought is the obsession and the act of throwing the salt is the compulsion or ritual. There are very few of us indeed who do not engage in some form of this superstitious behaviour. It may well go back to the days of magic, when an eclipse seemed to herald the end of the world, and complicated rituals were thought to protect families from the very real dangers that surrounded them. The difference between the superstition and a true obsessional disorder is that in the latter the thought repeats itself over and over, usually relieved only by another symbolic thought or act. Moreover, while I can manage *not* to touch wood or throw salt, an obsessional person cannot stop the ritual that provides relief. Between superstition and the obsessional-compulsive disorder – the real breakdown of control – lie those people who can be seen to have obsessional traits in their personalities, characterised by the 'houseproud woman' or the man who proudly describes himself as 'a perfectionist'.

The point at which an obsessional disorder might be diagnosed would usually be when anxious feelings are accompanied by disturbing, frightening or shameful thoughts which cannot be put out of your mind. This will often make you feel compelled to act in a certain way, either by some behaviour (like washing) or silently (like counting). At the same time you will be only too aware that thinking or acting like this has no sense to it and you'll battle constantly to stop. Neil described it in this way:

I have to start preparing for bed a couple of hours before I know it's time to sleep. Probably I'm thinking about it for quite a while before that. What happens is that I can't help myself checking and re-checking that I've locked up. I do it all very carefully, in the same order every night, going round all the windows and making sure the locks are tight, and then doing the same to all the doors. Then I usually do it again a couple of times before I actually go to bed, and I probably get up and do it two or three times more before I can get to sleep. I know it's ridiculous. I know on one level that I've checked and checked and that they must be secure, but I still have to go and do it again. My wife usually manages to reassure me enough for me to stop.

Lately I find I have a series of numbers that I count while I check, and it feels better if I get through them all perfectly. But so often I forget where I'm up to and so have to start again. Each time I finish I go through this battle trying to stop myself doing it all again, but I get dreadful thoughts about something awful happening to my family if I don't go through the whole routine.

Many obsessional thoughts concern harm coming to others; for example, that your spouse may have a dreadful accident driving home, or your child will drown whenever he or she goes swimming. Some of you may have frightening thoughts and images of causing the harm yourselves; for example, a mother may imagine herself hurling her baby out of the window or down the stairs, and develop some routine or ritual of other thoughts or behaviours in order to counteract it. Another group of obsessional thoughts may have to do with sexually obscene words or images. Perhaps the most common concern feelings of contamination – that you've been made dirty in some way – and these usually involve complicated routines of washing.

Ruth's obsessional thoughts and behaviours began shortly after she started working as a dental nurse. Although it was not really clear what her original fear was, she knew it was something to do with catching some awful disease and spreading it to her husband and children. She washed her hands dozens of times a day, and they were reddened and sore. She showered about three times a day with each one taking at least half an hour, and using up all the hot water each time. She would often get her husband to turn off the water so that she would have to come out. She used a couple of bottles of disinfectant a week around the house and in her car. There was a huge variety of things that she felt might have made her dirty; door handles, the sides of the sink, money, lavatories, bird droppings on the car, and so on.

Although there are links with dirt that we can all envisage in this list, other people may have less obvious cues that make them wash or perform some other ritual; for example, seeing a certain choco-late bar, or walking on cracks in the pavement or passing a particular street. Fears of harm may come from catching sight of a pair of scissors or a knife or a rope.

Obsessional thoughts are clearly distressing, but it's the compulsive acts that in the end cause the most problems in every-day life. For Ruth, she clearly was taking so much time in washing that she could no longer keep her job, and the cost of hot water and cleaning materials was a sore point to her husband. In Neil's case, he had little rest all evening, and it took a particularly patient wife to tolerate his constant checking. While a few people develop such extreme compulsions that they are literally unable to feed or look after themselves, others contain their problems in such a way that they can operate apparently normally, although they will usually appear somewhat withdrawn. This may be because they are going through complicated rituals in their heads, perhaps performing difficult mathematical calculations on car registrations, or digital clocks on videos, or account numbers. Although all this may sound quite mad, the person concerned *knows* that it's completely irrational and tries hard to resist, and this is why it's generally not regarded as psychotic.

Compared to most forms of psychological problems, obsessions are comparatively rare: probably not more than one person in 200 will suffer in this way. This may be an under-estimation, however, since very often people have their obsessions under enough control not to seek help. Although people with full obsessional disorders are usually very distressed by their symptoms, those with milder problems may see themselves as just being fussy: surely everyone checks their doors more than twice in this dangerous age, and so on. It seems somewhat ridiculous to say, well you have got a problem but you don't know it! Nevertheless, if you recognise any of these features in yourself or someone close, you can test if it's a problem by seeing if you can stop the thoughts or the actions. If this seems impossible then it's worth seeking some form of help.

The other complication in estimating the number of sufferers is that many of them may come to the doctor for depression or anxiety, and the obsession may be missed unless it is specifically raised as a problem by the patient. The importance of bringing it to light is that obsessions are much more easily cured in their early days, or at least when they do not present too much difficulty or disruption to a person's life.

WHAT CAUSES OBSESSIVE DISORDERS?

Very occasionally the start of an obsession is clear. Ann was a shy, rather quiet nine-year-old, the only child of restrained and somewhat cold parents. When, in 1962, the Cuban missile crisis occurred she remembers her teacher standing up in class to announce that there was a good chance of a nuclear war within the next 24 hours. Feeling terrified, sick and shaking, she went straight to her bedroom when she got home.

> *My parents thought I was poorly, I suppose, but actually I couldn't bear to hear the news. And over the next few weeks I got this conviction that if I heard the news we would all be destroyed – and, of course, it would be my fault! Sometimes I'd get engrossed in a book while my parents sat watching TV, and the news music would start and I'd have to leap up and hare upstairs with my fingers jammed in my ears. I honestly don't know if my parents ever noticed, but the Nine o'clock News still takes some watching. I bet there's lots of kids find it worse than a horror movie.*

Although Ann's case had an obvious beginning, there is perhaps less idea of what causes these problems than any other form of psychological disorder. It's clear, however, that the roots lie in anxiety: obsessive thoughts certainly seem to cause anxiety, but there is always the possibility that the anxiety is there already and the thoughts (for example, 'I might end up killing someone', or, 'My wife is enjoying obscene sexual acts with other men') are created almost to explain the pervading feeling of threat caused without apparent reason by the anxiety. This then would be an extreme form of the worrier who says, 'If I haven't got anything to worry about, I go and find something!' Certainly the ritual behaviours and thoughts – checking or counting or washing or whatever – seem to be done in order to reduce the awful feeling of anxiety and the thoughts that go with it.

One behavioural theory of cause proposes that fear was originally learnt to be associated with certain thoughts or objects, as in the development of phobias, which gradually generalised (became attached to more and more similar objects) over the years. Apart from occasional cases like Ann's there is little evidence for this, perhaps because the thought processes have become so elaborate by the time someone reaches therapy, that any origin has usually long ago been forgotten. However, quite a proportion of people seem to have experienced a life event, often a very stressful one, shortly before first noticing the symptoms. It is quite common for people to go through a brief period of obsessionality after some major life stress, perhaps as a way of experiencing an imaginary sense of control: but so long as it only lasts a few weeks it's not likely to be a problem.

Although the origins of the obsession may not be too clear, the behavioural reasons for the compulsions and rituals continuing are easier to understand. If you feel extreme anxiety at the sight of a Mars bar, and you by chance find that saying 'Fairy Liquid' to yourself reduces it (perhaps originally washing with Fairy reduced the feelings of contamination associated with the chocolate), it's quite likely that you'll go on saying it. When eventually it seems to lose some of its power, you might find that saying it three times works better. Each time you do it you are being rewarded by a reduction in anxiety, so no wonder you continue at all cost. We all know that most superstitions are ridiculous, but many of us go on doing them – just in case.

There is some evidence for cognitive theories which suggest that if you are suffering from an obsession you may well have unusually high expectations of bad outcomes. Certainly Neil, described above, was abnormally pessimistic about all manner of things, not just being broken into and attacked. Throughout his work as a civil engineer he would raise problems that no one else would consider remotely possible. At the same time, although they joked about this way of overestimating the chance of something going wrong, his colleagues managed to value it as well, and the firm's excellent reputation may well have been helped by Neil's voice of gloom.

Other evidence for a basis to the disorder linked to the way you think comes from research showing that obsessional people have a greater need of certainty and are more perfectionist. Although these traits are fine for some jobs where checking is important, they can destroy careers in certain occupations. For example, I once knew a doctor who took his patients' temperatures three or four times in every consultation; felt their pulses over and over; and even ran down the road after them to check their colour once again. Of course, nothing amiss escaped him and in that sense he was an excellent doctor, but trying to run a general practice with such a problem was obviously extremely distressing, and eventually impossible.

Certainly obsessional people seem to be of slightly higher intelligence than the average person. There is, however, little evidence that genetic factors play a role in causing the disorder. Parents and brothers and sisters of sufferers are slightly more likely to show obsessional problems than those unrelated in this way, but if some of the personality features of rigidity, perfectionism and pessimism are part of the family culture, they're likely to be picked up from each other rather than inherited. Living with someone with an obsessional disorder can be extremely stressful, and so quite likely to produce some form of psychological problem in other family members.

TREATMENTS

Like all psychological problems, you can't just tell a person who's going through some form of obsessional-compulsive disorder simply to pull themselves together. One of the central aspects of the breakdown is that they know that everything they're doing is irrational and they are trying very hard to resist their actions, but can't. Similarly, reassurance may actually make things worse, so it's always better to stop reassuring and to convince the person to go for help. In the early stages, self-help may be possible and should be tackled using the behavioural strategies outlined below.

Basically the two aspects that need tackling in treatment are the anxiety that is connected with the obsessional thoughts, and the 'rewards' (through reducing anxiety) that are provided by the compulsive behaviours. By far the most useful way of doing this comes from behaviour therapy and most professionals in the field would choose this as an essential part of treatment.

As a way of stopping the compulsive rituals which take up so much time for sufferers and which are so disruptive of family and work, Meyer, a British psychologist, devised a procedure of repeatedly making the person face whatever causes the discomfort (Mars bars, the news, dog-muck, unlocked doors, knives, and so on) for longer and longer periods, usually building up from situations that cause the least problem to those that cause the most. This procedure takes place 10 to 20 times a day, and they are asked not to do whatever they would normally be compelled to do – wash, or check or count, for example. At the same time the helper will probably model the procedure himself or herself, but not give the patient any reassurance as to safety, etc.

About three-quarters of people are helped by this treatment, and both Neil and Ruth did well using it. Neil's psychologist worked with him in his home with the help of his wife, but Ruth was admitted to hospital for a few days so that the treatment regime could be carried out more intensively.

About three weeks before I went in, my psychologist taught me a form of relaxation. I found it pretty impossible for a while, and how much I actually used it during the treatment I'm not really sure. But I find I use it more and more often now and it's wonderful. It's just hard to remember how well I used it during the treatment. Then we agreed a list of objects and situations that would make me wash. I think it went from the inside of the bathroom sink through to touching bird-droppings, with dozens of other things in between. Shaking hands with people was about half way up, I remember. One of the problems was that, once outside I couldn't be sure that birds hadn't gone on anything that I might touch, and so touching walls, trees, the grass and pavements all had to fit into the hierarchy. It was an embarrassingly long list by the time we'd finished it!

Anyway, in hospital I had a wonderful nurse therapist assigned to me. She was ever so patient, but also very firm. We started at the sink. First I had to touch the part closest to where the water went down, and then gradually touch more and more towards the rim and outside, which I found more bothersome. I desperately wanted to wash but she took me to have a cup of tea. This became the pattern – working higher and higher up the hierarchy, not washing and gradually eating meals straight afterwards without washing my hands. She was very good at spotting some of my less obvious ways of avoiding things, like not sitting properly on park benches, just on the edge in case I was sitting in something nasty! She came back home with me and we ran through bits of the hierarchy again, making me touch my husband and children after I'd touched a door-knob or shaken hands, for example.

After this I was given exercises to do on my own, making sure I kept on touching things and not washing. Ray, my husband, was not allowed to reassure me at all (which he'd always done before), but he was really good at making sure I kept up with the exercises. We went on lots of picnics, and he'd forget to take a rug deliberately so I'd have to sit on the grass. Things like that.

Sometimes, after considerable success, you may slip back a bit, or perhaps find a new obsession. It's important not to regard this as a failure, but to start again to tackle it in the same way. Usually you will manage to control things better each time. For those of you who have spent hours a day on your rituals, it's important that some more fulfilling activity is planned, even before you start treatment. Otherwise, life may actually seem a bit empty!

The obsessional thoughts themselves often reduce without being specifically tackled: they did in Ruth's case. Sometimes strategies are given to stop them, such as distracting yourself with something else, or shouting STOP! to yourself each time they come, at first out loud and later just in your head. Neil found these methods weren't enough to stop him worrying about harm coming to his family, although he had managed to stop checking the locks each night. He therefore was given more exploratory psychotherapy to look at the meaning of his underlying anxiety, and this proved very helpful.

There is no doubt that suffering from this disorder is very disturbing of life and very depressing for the sufferers. For this reason you will often be given minor tranquillisers or an antidepressant drug, at least to help with the anxiety and depressive symptoms. There is no evidence that tranquillisers do help, but there are reports suggesting that one particular antidepressant, clomipramine, has an effect on the obsessional symptoms as well as the depression. However, these improvements are short-lived once the drug is stopped, and so it's always better to have behavioural treatment alongside any drugs.

There is also some evidence that, in extreme cases, psychosurgery (leucotomy or lobotomy) reduces the worst of the symptoms. However, this is a very extreme form of treatment and, because so few are carried out, its effects (especially the long-term effects) are far from clear. For this reason, if used at all, it should only ever be a last resort when all other forms of therapy have been tried. In addition I would always recommend trying more than one therapist as well as different therapies, because we're all a bit different, even if we seem to be applying the same methods, and one person will respond better to one therapist than another.

As an example of this, I once witnessed a woman cured by a very junior trainee psychologist. She had suffered from the disorder very seriously for many years and, after numerous treatment attempts, was considering psychosurgery. He had noticed during a ward-round that she was hyperventilating (p. 46), and taught her that the resulting lack of carbon dioxide was causing anxiety symptoms which she then labelled as caused by fears about her family. By *re*-labelling her anxiety as the consequence of over-breathing, and then learning how to breathe more normally, she managed to reduce her symptoms considerably and, after further behavioural treatment, was eventually discharged from hospital. I don't want to say there's always an answer like this – there isn't – but to encourage people to really explore every avenue before deciding that their problems are so intolerable that they are willing to consider psychosurgery.

OBSESSIONAL PERSONALITIES

At the beginning of the chapter I mentioned people who seem to have obsessional traits in their personalities: those who can be termed perfectionists, who become upset at the crumpled cushion, the uncut lawn, the scuffed shoe, or the impunctual guest. Even the most untidy of us often have a little corner of this tucked away in the rest of the chaos: the man whose rooms are a wealth of dusty jumble but whose stamp collection shows the meticulous cataloguing of a fanatic. But for many of us the experience of chaos, mess, complexity will cause good resolutions, even the possibility of activity to change things for the better, but no real anxiety.

For the obsessional personality such disorder is distressing, and needs to be immediately corrected. It does not usually produce the compulsive behaviours discussed above, but an uncontrollable change in the rigid routine of life may instead bring about anxiety in the short term, and depression if the change continues.

Jonathon was referred by his doctor for psychotherapy after he sought help for the depression he'd experienced since being promoted. He was not sure if it was the job itself, or whether he was still feeling guilty about his constant irritability that had occurred lately and which had led him, for the first time in their marriage, to strike his wife. He came over as pretty irritable to his therapist too: he told her within the first few sessions and in no uncertain terms that he really held no truck with all this psychological nonsense, and that, if he was going to go to an expert, he wished he'd been sent to a man.

His therapist said she thought he sounded pretty angry and he loudly declared, thumping the arm of the chair, that of course he wasn't angry, but would she please get on with whatever they had to do; he hated all this hanging about and he couldn't bear the silences. She suggested to him that perhaps what was most difficult was the uncertainty of what was happening: that nothing in therapy seemed clear-cut and definite; that there were no facts. At this his anxiety became undeniable and could no longer be covered up with anger. She made a link to his new job: he'd left the concreteness of columns of figures and definite outcomes, where each day had a rigid routine and was on the whole predictable, and been promoted to a job that called for a flexible approach.

Many people who live rigidly (for example, who take the same newspaper every day because taking something with a less fixed party-line would feel like inviting chaos and anarchy into their lives) often feel that any step outside this straight-jacket of a life would open the floodgates to something they fear but cannot name. In Jonathon's case, this nameless messy unacknowledged area was his rage. The uncertainty of his new job had prodded it into the open in a burst against his wife, and, although he'd put the lid back on as well as he could, it still kept bubbling out at his therapist and to people at work and at home. The whole experience had put him in touch with the uncertainty and ultimate uncontrollability of life – a difficult experience for most of us and one for which Jonathon had developed no coping strategies and no philosophy since he'd spent so much of his life making sure things were controllable and predictable.

I guess in the end the most important part of therapy for me was eventually just letting myself experience all the uncertainty and complexity of the therapy and of myself. All the time at the beginning I wanted to run away from it – to have someone give me some simple exercises rather than encourage me to get into the mess. Definitely acknowledging my anger and getting an idea of where it arose and that, for a child, it had been quite justifiable but forbidden, that was all really helpful. I still catch myself wishing everything was simple and controllable, but now I can just about accept that it isn't – that I can't control everything in my life. It's terribly difficult at first, and then it's just such a relief!

Chapter

Eating problems

A woman can never be too rich or too thin.

(Duchess of Windsor)

*My fat says 'screw you' to all who want me to be the perfect mom,
sweetheart, maid and whore . . .*

(Susie Orbach)

It is hard to view that beautiful slender young woman, smiling
and attentive, as having any kind of nervous breakdown. Her
elegant layers of clothing make you sure you've seen her in Vogue.
If you're a man you may well give her an appreciative glance, and
if you're a woman you'll probably experience at least a tinge of
envy. If a nervous breakdown means that something has gone out
of control and can't easily be mended by the individual concerned,
then surely this woman represents the very opposite: surely
anyone who can control their eating so efficiently and exercise so
regularly that they can look like this, can't have any problems?

And yet, if this young woman continues her bizarre pattern of
eating into the future you both may change your opinions. You
may realise the chaos of her mind as you watch her become so thin
that her joints stand out from limbs that are literally skin and
bones; you'll see her face become skull-like and covered with fine
'lagunal' hair; and if you dare to hug her, you may well crack her

ribs. Not a pretty sight at all, but also only one step away from the media image of the perfect woman.

There are three categories of eating problems in the psychiatric diagnostic system, and the vast majority of sufferers are women. **Anorexia nervosa** is characterised by constant dieting; **compulsive eating**, involves gorging massive quantities of food at one sitting, and so results in becoming overweight; and **bulimia** is a combination of compulsive eating followed by vomiting or purging.

ANOREXIA NERVOSA

Anorexia means a loss of appetite, and nervosa suggests that this is due to psychological rather than physical causes. However, now that the real experiences of these women have at last been listened to, it is clear that there is absolutely no loss of appetite. They are literally starving and, like all starving people, they are obsessed unendingly with the thought of food. Over the past decade this disorder has attracted enormous attention in the press, and especially in women's magazines, and many self-help groups and women's therapy services have specialised in this and other eating problems. But the numbers never seem to dwindle.

Anorexia nervosa can occur at any age, but by far the majority of sufferers are in their adolescence, with over 90 per cent being female. As puberty begins earlier each decade, so it seems does anorexia. Although it's usually easy for parents to notice that their young daughter's food intake has dwindled, it is more difficult later in adolescence when young women are able to be more secretive and when, in any case, it is the norm to diet: one study showed that by the age of 17, 70 to 80 per cent of girls are trying to lose weight, even though very few of these are actually fat. In fact anorexia may be much less of a problem if people – sufferers and parents – would seek help sooner. But they don't. Perhaps partly because they're both conforming to the media norm of the angular female, and also because of the desperate refusal of the girl herself to admit that she is anything but healthy, they often get down to 35–50 kg (and occasionally considerably less) before they or someone close to them finally seeks help. The scheming to resist a cure, even when it's offered, by means of extra layers of clothes, hiding of food, secreting weights on themselves when they are weighed, and so on, has a deviousness matched only by alcoholics and other addicts.

It's not just young women and those close to them who may ignore the fact that dieting has become out of control; professionals are also subject to the same stereotypes of slimness and so may also miss the condition, as Helena describes:

I'd been very overweight for a couple of years. I think I was pretty fed up at the time. Then I decided to diet. I lost weight quite quickly and people noticed straight away. They really started treating me different as I got slimmer. I felt they had more respect for me. I reached the weight I'd been when I got married within about three months, but I wanted to go on. From then on I know (although I'd have denied it completely at the time) that I began to say I wasn't dieting any more; I'd tell them how I ate like a pig but just didn't get fat. All that kind of thing. In fact I lived on spinach, celery and the odd egg, and if people came to dinner I'd eat nearly the same as them and then go and make myself sick. But that wasn't very often. I dropped in all from twelve stone to just above seven. I kept it about there mainly because I'm tall and because I really couldn't eat any less. I swam a mile every day. People said I looked wonderful, but I still saw myself as overweight.

She and her husband decided it was time to start a family. Her periods had stopped a few months before, but she didn't take much notice; it just meant she had to keep on having pregnancy tests because they could never be sure if she was pregnant or not. Nothing happened. Not surprising, because when you diet heavily and your periods stop, it's usually an indication that you're no longer ovulating. After about a year they started going to a sterility clinic where, missing that this was an eating problem, the doctors put her on a course of injections to encourage ovulation. It was only two miserable years later when nothing had happened that a new woman doctor at the local practice saw Helena as anorexic. She was referred (with great reluctance on her part) to an eating disorders group at a woman's therapy centre and, since her weight had never gone critically low, she was helped quite soon to look at herself and her eating habits. With weight gain her periods began once more and she conceived shortly after.

So apart from a painfully low intake of food, these young women are also characterised by long arduous exercise of one sort or another, amenorrhoea (or the end of periods), and a distorted perception which makes them see their emaciated body as repulsively overweight. This misperception actually becomes less as they put on weight once more. In boys the pattern is similar, usually beginning soon after puberty, with excessive dieting and exercise, and a reduction of male hormones and their newly acquired interest in sex.

Occasionally this disorder is called 'slimmer's disease'. This is extremely unhelpful, because it suggests that the girl or boy has some physical abnormality which reduces the desire for food. In fact, there is no evidence of any physical cause to anorexia (though undoubtedly physical changes other than the obvious weight loss are likely to occur as a result of it) and, as we said above, these people rarely lose their desire for food.

One of the findings concerning anorexia nervosa, as opposed to the other eating disorders, is that sufferers are predominantly from the middle classes, and it is quite likely that the middle-class philosophy of achievement, competition, and deferred gratification (putting off getting good experiences now in order to gain later success) is a perfect one to foster this behaviour.

One theory about cause comes from the fact that the main time for the disorder to begin occurs at or shortly after puberty, and also that there are often unacknowledged problems in the parents' marriage and in the family as a whole. Salvador Minuchin's work has found that the parents of young anorexic women are often over-protective and rather rigidly unchanging. They avoid conflict at any cost, and have been described as 'enmeshed', so the family as a whole is paramount and there is little chance for individual expression or change in any one of them. It is suggested that such a family makes it very difficult for the turbulence, separation and change of adolescence to take place. The sudden fierce dieting routine returns the girl to a pre-puberty state with her periods ceasing and her newly acquired hips and breasts vanishing. The threat to the family that was caused by the daughter's sexuality is therefore removed by the anorexia and, it is suggested, this may be one reason why some parents take so long before they decide that she needs help.

The link between sex and eating is discussed by Annie Fursland in her chapter in *Fed Up and Hungry*. She points out that it's remained with us ever since Eve met the serpent, and is as strong as ever today. For example, we talk of being 'wicked' in over-eating, and adverts tell us that huge gooey cream cakes are 'naughty, but nice', while others use double meanings to joke about butter and having an exceptional appetite for sex. People who eat a lot and are overweight are considered to have no self-restraint: they 'stuff' themselves. Apart from stopping food-intake in an unconscious attempt to stop their sexuality, young women who see sex as immoral may well see food as immoral too.

Whereas men are said to have 'healthy appetites' (both in their eating habits and in their sexual urges), women are frowned on for this. I remember one manfriend I had while still a student: I had noticed on several occasions that, whenever we went out to dinner and I cleared my plate (which I always did due to my chronic lack of money), he appeared to sulk for some time afterwards. One day when, due to a bilious attack, I left half my food, he looked pleased and told me he hated women who ate heartily: they were sloppy and had too little control, and anyway, it appeared to him that they were enjoying their food more than his company! Over a young lifetime, innumerable signs of criticism from parents, friends and lovers, at any hint of excess, are received and regis-tered, if not always remembered.

The other problem of these over-protective, enmeshed families is that they do not allow the children to control aspects of their lives. As the American writer, Hilde Bruch, points out, they may have the mothers who say, 'I'm cold, put your jumper on', or 'I'm hungry; we'll eat now', or 'I'm wide awake, so I brought you a cup of tea'. When the parents finally bring their daughter for help she is usually described as being very good and obedient: she's been hard-working at school and always done everything they've told her. Rebellion takes place via the socially acceptable means of dieting – at last they have an area of their lives they can control. While this is extremely powerful (hunger strike has been used by protesters of all sorts, especially this century), it is also self-destructive and so ultimately useless.

Although research has shown that these types of family relation-ships appear in many cases of anorexia nervosa, not all sufferers start so young or have such upbringings. A far larger factor that they have in common is that the vast majority are women, and any discussion of cause must take this into account. Families are a product of society and family pressures reflect society's pressures.

Already we have seen some relevant differences between the sexes which take place in the family: girls are more protected than boys; their puberty poses more threat (we have 'fallen women' but never 'fallen men'); their appetites are subtly more controlled. Society as a whole has a constant effect on women's attitude to themselves and on men's attitude to them by dictating the shape that they should be. Whereas in past centuries rich men wanted their women fat to distinguish them from the thin and starving poor, now that everyone in the West has 'sufficient' food, the mark of a rich woman becomes her thinness, as the quote from the Duchess of Windsor illustrates.

Since the sixties the media dictates on fashionable shape have gone so far as to make women look as much as possible like men. They should lose their female attributes of rounded belly and full hips and thighs, and take on the male shape, hipless and narrow thighs. One woman who became anorexic in her thirties described her bewilderment:

> When I was a teenager I could never reach the weight they said I should be. I was 5' 4" and I should have weighed nine stone three according to all the charts. I really used to try to fatten myself up, but it wasn't till I'd had a couple of kids that I began to fill out. By that time the charts had changed completely. Now I should be not much more than eight stone, and models were obviously a lot less than that. It felt that I was always trying to be what they wanted and, just as I'd get close they'd change the rules. I should have said, 'Who cares?' but I didn't. I cared very much indeed and so I began to diet, and it became the most important thing in my life. And there I was: four and a half stone; scared stiff of dying, but terrified of putting on an ounce!

The 64-billion-dollar question is why women follow fashion at all – why they let others dictate their insides and outsides in this way, and why some will die rather than follow their bodies' natural messages. One reason, put forward by both feminist therapists and by psychological research, is that women don't like themselves too much. Increasingly over their childhood they see themselves as inferior to others, as less intelligent, less attractive, less competent, and so on. Research shows that if they fail at school they will blame this on a lack of brains, whereas boys will blame their teacher or their laziness (something which can be changed). Even now they are brought up as second-class citizens and still, in many families, the male members are given the largest and choicest of the food. Most women, not just those with anorexia, are more likely nowadays to perceive themselves as overweight.

So they struggle on with their endless, ever-changing target of media-created perfection. Whereas once they changed their bodies as society dictated by binding their feet or whittling their waists with corsets or elongating their necks with umpteen rings, now they can do it by diet alone. Their targets appear in every newspaper, magazine and television programme; whereas the photos of newsworthy men may be fat, old, balding, but are invariably powerful, photos of women are predominantly slim, beautiful and often without a role.

There is no doubt that anorexia nervosa, like all psychological disorders, has no single cause but reflects a number of aspects. The pressures and restrictions created by both families and society as a whole may precipitate you into dieting. The diet is rewarded quickly by people's reactions to you – you have such self-control, you look so good (that is, like the current fashion), you're envied and respected. These opinions are both novel and gratifying and not easy to give up, and so the dieting continues. At some point it's possible that physical changes take place: certainly the misconceptions of your body-size get larger as you become thinner. You're on the wrong road, and so the search is endless.

Treatments for anorexia nervosa are largely psychological. Though you may be depressed, prescribing antidepressant drugs is rarely useful since your low mood generally lifts once you gain some weight. There is therefore usually a period when the main effort of treatment is aimed at getting you back to a safe weight, especially if you've grown so thin that your life is threatened. This will inevitably involve hospitalisation, and usually bedrest until the target weight is achieved. Occasionally sufferers are fed intravenously (through a tube straight into the bloodstream), but at least they are likely to find initially that all their meals and visits to the bathroom are supervised.

This can be a pretty dreadful period. For a start you will have a really deep terror of putting on weight: weight signifies something to be ashamed of, the mark of self-indulgence, social failure and condemnation by others. Lisa was 17 when she went into hospital:

I was 37 kg. They wanted me to agree that I would reach 45, but I couldn't bear to think of being so big. It filled me with panic. I came to an agreement that I would get up to 41, but in fact once I was there the panic wasn't so awful, and I was actually 51 kg when I was discharged.

In some hospitals this encouragement for weight gain is done on behavioural lines: giving rewards (such as being able to get up and watch TV) and taking them away depending on the direction of the change. Since one aspect of anorexia is the urge for self-determination – the need to control one aspect of life efficiently – this apparent taking away of all control may not seem the most appropriate remedy in the long run. A gain in weight is obviously essential, but can usually be achieved without such coercion by building up a trusting relationship with one of the nurses who is experienced in the anguish that the young girl will initially feel.

Although it is not so difficult to achieve a weight gain by these methods, if this is the extent of the treatment the chances of relapse are quite high. A proportion of people who are in one way or another simply force-fed are quite likely to turn to vomiting rather than dieting as a means of weight loss and, if this occurs, the hopes of final cure become smaller. Therefore once a reasonable gain has been achieved, most hospitals will begin some form of psychotherapy to explore the origins of your dieting, perhaps going into some of the difficulties in the family relationships. This will usually begin in hospital and carry on as an outpatient when you leave. If your periods don't begin with a return to normal weight, hormone treatment can be given to start them again.

If the weight loss is not too substantial, anorexia nervosa will usually be treated by a psychiatrist or psychologist in an outpatient clinic, sometimes simply by setting targets. This should be especially possible in a young girl or boy where the parents have been prompt in seeking help. If this is not the first time the problem has occurred psychotherapy may be offered, or, where the child is still young and at home, the whole family may be asked to attend for family therapy.

Family therapy is particularly successful where young people are involved. It follows the idea that a family is a system of interlocking parts. The problem is seen as lying not in one or other individual within it, but in the family as a whole. This means that if you change any part of the system – for example, by changing a thin pre-sexual child into a healthy autonomous young woman – all the other parts of the system simply have to change in some way: there is just no way things can be the same again. Like all change, this can be quite scary, but also very liberating as family members become less rigid and explore new ways of operating. The first change may not come from the child, but perhaps from a parent behaving in a less intrusive or over-protected manner, as Marilyn points out:

When the psychologist first suggested family therapy, Paul and I became really angry. We'd brought Jill for help which she clearly needed, and it felt as if the spotlight was being shifted from her to us. Looking back I can see I'd already been feeling pretty guilty about Jill's weight loss, and suggesting the family was the patient made me more guilty, which of course made me angry! I'm pretty sure Paul felt the same. The psychologist made us all sit down to lunch together for a start, and watched how we operated in trying to get Jill to eat something. He made some pretty useful comments straight away, and then asked me to try eating without watching Jill or speaking to her about her food: as he pointed out, that had done no good whatsoever, so we needed to find another way. Both Paul and I found this exercise made us feel incredibly anxious – far more so than when we concentrated on Jill.

Doing this gradually let us realise we needed to look at other issues in the family, and particularly at our marriage. Pressures burst out that had been sat upon for years. We often felt like never going again, but we always went and really it was exciting in the end and both of us, and the girls, are getting on so much better. We'd got stuck in something and didn't dare to move. I think we thought that if we did change, the whole family and marriage would crumble. In fact, the reverse was true.

Over the past 10 years another important form of therapy for anorexia has developed, springing from the women's movement and the fact that it is predominantly women who suffer from eating disorders. Many of the ideas behind this came from Susie Orbach's book, *Fat is a Feminist Issue*, published in the late seventies, which looked more at compulsive eating, but had important implications for anorexia. Feminist therapists use traditional forms of group and individual psychotherapy but do not overlook the reality of society's pressures on women and how much these have increased this century until we have the Superwoman image of the eighties where the perfect woman is successful in education, in a career, as a mother, a lover – and, of course, is slim. Various women's therapy centres have begun around the country. Most are under-funded and over-subscribed, but the women who've attended and whom I've talked to have had nothing but good words for their experience.

Many of these centres organise, or will put you in touch with, self-help groups, though these are not always suitable for fully anorexic women since they can too easily develop into competitive slimming unless the dieting behaviour has actually ceased.

BULIMIA

Deborah describes her experiences:

> *I'd been teaching at the same school for the past four years. I got on well with the children and the staff seemed to think I was OK, probably because I appeared such a hard worker. I don't suppose they would have described me as either thin or fat, but I always thought of myself as overweight. One thing was for sure: no one knew what went into keeping me just this size. Around mid-afternoon I might think, 'I've done well today; I've been so busy that I've missed lunch.' Although this was deliberate, I'd pretend it wasn't and that I wasn't really hungry. I'd decide, as I did on most days, that this must be a good day to start a diet. But then something would go wrong – I'd feel I must ring my mother or my sister or something and everything would go cold and empty.*
>
> *I'd drive as fast as I could to the huge anonymous supermarket near the school. I might buy a couple of large loaves of Mother's Pride, three chocolate cakes, a pack of Mars bars, a couple of pints of milk. Basically a large pile of carbohydrate. Anonymous or not, I'd feel terrified the woman at the till would know what I did with food. I had an hour and a half before John was due home. Inside my house I'd sit down and stuff and stuff till I couldn't fit any more in and then I'd stick my toothbrush handle down my throat and vomit it all back up. I would feel disgusting and depressed, and hate myself for having such a ghastly secret.*

Deborah is suffering from bulimia or bulimia nervosa or buli-marexia. Whichever name it's given it describes a disorder where the main method of weight control is by vomiting or occasionally by taking huge doses of laxatives, or abusing diuretics or thyroid-containing preparations. There's nothing new about vomiting after over-indulgence: the Romans did it often, and it may be an efficient way, once a year after the office party, to feel better the next morning. But in bulimia, really enormous quantities of highly fattening food are consumed at one sitting, but never with any enjoyment; it may happen weekly or as often as several times a day. Although again most sufferers are women, now it's becoming increasingly discussed, it's clear that there are also a large number of men with the disorder.

Often it begins out of severe anorexia, sometimes after patients have been fed up to a desired weight but given no appropriate therapy to look at the causes of their fasting. But these are the rather more public examples of bulimia, those already on the record as anorexics. We cannot estimate how many others there are – those women and men who never diet long term, and who may be thin, average or even overweight – since bulimia is above all a secret activity.

It's also a dangerous activity: persistent vomiting or purging causes a serious loss of your body fluids and a reduction of potassium levels. It can lead to urinary infections and epileptic seizures, and death is possible in severe cases. The other danger is suicide, since bulimic men and women have none of the pride of those with anorexia who are, after all, only going one step beyond the demands set by society. These people despise and disgust themselves constantly by their behaviour, both aspects of which are socially frowned upon, especially in a world where half the people are starving. The guilt and self-hate this induces makes suicide a real risk.

Treatment may begin with hospitalisation to restore you to a pattern of normal eating. There may also be a behavioural programme to get you to learn which situations or relationships prompt the bouts of stuffing, and to help you to work out suitable strategies to overcome the anxiety that these situations create. In addition, psychotherapy, whether through in- and out-patient services, or a women's therapy centre, will probably look at the bulimia as a symptom and symbol of some deeper distress which made you dislike yourself so deeply and makes you so ambivalent about being nourished or loved.

This was the path taken by Deborah. She was in a pretty

desperate state, both physically and psychologically, when she finally went to her doctor. In hospital she was kept on the ward, away from the hospital shop and its temptations, and given food only at mealtimes. She was put on a course of antidepressants since it was clear to the psychiatrist that she was feeling pretty wretched by then. A behavioural nurse therapist worked with her during this time, teaching her to recognise what made her anxious and long to stuff, and ways to cope with this anxiety. The clear message came from this, that it was phone calls to or from her mother and, to a lesser extent, her sister, that were prime causes for this anxiety.

On discharge she found that she was coping better than before by using relaxation and avoiding phoning her mother in situations where she could easily get hold of food, and using the cognitive strategies her therapist had taught her. But despite her boyfriend's help in all this she also felt pretty alone and terrified of slipping back. A friend recommended a woman psychologist who worked privately in the town. At Deborah's protests, she pointed out that it seemed easier to pay for vast quantities of rubbish food that she would throw up at once, than to pay for therapy that would help. So Deborah, reluctantly, went. It was a difficult, long, slow process; partly because, as she couldn't hang on to nourishment, so too she found it difficult to hang on to the good things from therapy. She'd chuck them away angrily, turn up late, forget appointments, and so on. But gradually as she understood how much this reflected the way her mother, an alcoholic, had treated her – giving her smothering love and then ferocious anger; giving her toys and then selling them for drink – then she began to see and make sense of her eating and gradually the dreadful urges left her.

The important message is that however tired you are of dieting, don't start vomiting or purging as a way round it. Tackle the reason you have chosen to diet: that's what's important. If you are already locked into this cycle, then do seek help. Just knowing there are many like you on its own reduces the loneliness and the despair. Of course change is difficult, but it's also very possible.

COMPULSIVE EATING

Around one in 20 men and one in nine women in Britain are overweight by at least 20 per cent. How many of these eat compulsively – that is, gorging vast, uncomfortable quantities of food at one sitting – is not known. While being overweight alone is hardly criteria for having a nervous breakdown, compulsive eating, usually conducted secretly, is often accompanied by depression, irritability and restlessness. In the western world, the fat person is a figure of fun, and as such he or she either has to be comic or there is very little acceptance of them.

The compulsive eating side of obesity is similar to that in bulimia, except that you won't be vomiting at the end of a session. Chances are however, that you'll feel pretty disgusted and ashamed and make all sorts of vows to yourself that you'll never do it again.

Many of us eat for comfort, and compulsive eating often takes place during stressful periods of our lives: rows with your spouse, children leaving home, difficulties at work, and so on. Inside we feel 'empty' and scared, and we fill this emptiness with food when maybe all we need is love. Some of us perhaps came from homes where everyone was overweight, where food was given when a cuddle may have been more appropriate. But there is another side to compulsive eating: some of us do it to show the world (or someone in particular) that we'll not conform to their rules, that we'll not be what they want. As Jacob said:

Every time I visit home, I see my parents looking at me with this sad worried little look that makes me so furious. It's saying, 'Oh, Jacob, how are you ever going to get a nice girlfriend and get married and give us grandchildren when you look so horribly, disgustingly fat?' It makes me have second helpings of everything on the table, and then carve myself a huge plate of sandwiches when we've finished!

There is clearly often a lot of anger underlying some obesity, probably because it's not expressed. One client I saw, Alison, had given up her own academic career when she married her husband and concentrated on his. She cared for his every need, sitting up late at night to help him with his statistics, explain the significance of his results, and finally type up his thesis, while hers lay dusty in a box. When he was given a lectureship and a research grant, she became his assistant (at the same time as looking after their children and doing all the housework and cooking). All this and never a cross word! But she ate and ate. He clearly hated her huge fatness and was always bringing home new diets for her to try. But she'd sneak down in the middle of the night and have a loaf of bread and a packet of Weetabix.

It wasn't difficult to reduce Alison's weight; just getting her to keep a diary of what she ate each day made her lose two stone in a few weeks. Analysing the situations in which she ate gave her ways to change her behaviour. But it was obviously very important that I kept on looking at the diary; she was doing it for my approval, not for her own good, and if I didn't make enough fuss of what she'd done, she'd have a binge. This often shows in research – a behavioural regime for obesity is most successful if the therapist uses a periodic follow-up at least by phone, just to see how the client is getting on. It's also why Weight Watchers works best if you're a life member!

I tackled this issue with Alison, and she agreed she needed approval desperately. No matter what she gave up for her husband, he never seemed satisfied. 'But', I suggested, 'You won't give up your weight for him.' 'Why should I?' roared Alison, and then apologised for shouting. It was the first time I'd really seen the anger, though I'd suspected it was there when she binged if I didn't praise her. Rather than apologise for it, we encouraged it to really let rip within the therapy. No, they didn't live happily ever after. But, yes she did resume her studies, lose several stone, and have a good relationship with her children.

That fat can have a purpose, especially for women, was a theory put forward by Orbach in *Fat is a Feminist Issue*. This book provided enormous relief to countless women who had struggled, whether by the ways described in this chapter, or simply by the yearly diet, to be what society demanded. Out of the book came a network of self-help groups which can be very successful for compulsive eating in particular. But its underlying message, appropriate for men and women alike, is to learn to trust and listen to your body. To hear it when it says it's hungry and to pay attention when it says it's had enough. This way you won't start on any of the desperate paths to nowhere described above.

Chapter

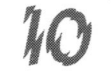

Alcohol and addiction

When Guy's second marriage broke up, he was forced to sell his house and move to a small rented flat on the other side of town. He knew no one, but could not bear the new loneliness of his evenings, and so went to the pub each night at eight. There, within a few days, he had met three or four other regulars with whom he could natter. Although he would have preferred to space his drinks, he could see that it was important to these men that he drank 'with them', pint for pint. During the day he was a salesman heading his own team and doing very well at it. Of course, there had always been a lot of necessary socialising there too: drinks with the customers over expense-account lunches, and drinks with the team after work. Now he lived alone he just had time for fish and chips before he headed for the local.

I really didn't think I drank an excessive amount; perhaps because the settings were so different I could stick them into separate compartments, and not bother to add up what I was drinking over 24 hours. I rarely felt drunk: maybe the odd Saturday night when I'd carry through from lunchtime till final closing, but not during the week. But I did begin to feel pretty desperate in the mornings. I'd often wake around four or five, feeling ghastly: not just nauseous, but hands shaking, and tense and irritable. I knew a drink made the feelings go away, and I'd have a stiff whisky as soon as I got to the office, but incredibly I still didn't let myself see the connection. I even went to my GP with it and, because I'd been through such a rough time with my marriage and everything, he thought I was suffering from anxiety and feeling a bit depressed. Not surprising really, because I'd told him I only drank a couple of pints a night. I almost believed it myself! He gave me some Valium and told me I shouldn't drink while I was taking them. Well, I managed that all right for a few days. Felt quite virtuous, even. Then the pleasure from that vanished and I found myself drinking hard again.

Over the next year I lost my licence and got into a couple of fights. Finally my boss hauled me in and said my work was going down fast, people had complained about me, and if I didn't do something about my drinking straight away I'd be out of a job. In a way it was a relief. Someone had said 'stop' at last. The works doctor sent me to a counsellor and, after some individual work, she introduced me to this group. When I think of how close being in a good job and having a bit of prestige is to being on skid row I come out in a cold sweat. If I'd lost my job I really think I'd be there by now.

Guy typifies many addicts in the way his addictive behaviour (in his case drinking) progressed. He did it regularly and daily and made sure he was always prepared with drink (just as a smoker makes sure he or she always has cigarettes). Alcohol made him 'normal', not necessarily drunk, and in periods when he stopped he became tense and irritable and, like any heroin addict, suffered physiological withdrawal effects as well. Although he was excellent at denying it, he knew he felt compelled to drink – just as compulsive gamblers go on for a long time declaring it's just a hobby, but on another level are aware they can no longer control the activity. Like most addictions he needed more and more to gain the same effect.

That problem drinking is an addiction with the same pattern of compulsive, self-destructive behaviour as gambling, compulsive eating, flashing, smoking, drug abuse, and even jogging, is an argument put forward by Heather and Robertson in their book *Problem Drinking: The New Approach.* Certainly there are clear similarities between the various behaviours, and for this reason and because it is the most widespread addictive behaviour, we are only considering problems with alcohol in this chapter. If you have another addiction you will undoubtedly see the links with your own behaviour – if you are finally able to acknowledge your problems – and the bibliography and address list will provide more specific help.

The terms 'alcoholic' and 'alcoholism', which imply that you are suffering from a disease, are far less frequently used nowadays. More common is the term 'problem drinker' which covers, first, those who may not be addicted to alcohol, but who are suffering from its effects – financially, legally, socially or in their health; and second, those who are addicted, or 'alcohol dependent', those like Guy who would have difficulty giving up drinking and who suffer physical effects when they try to do so.

Alcohol is so much a part of our lives in terms of social interactions, business deals, and leisure-time activities, that it may be hard for most of us to see problem drinking as being in any real sense a nervous breakdown. Certainly the breakdown is not dramatic: heavy drinkers may have physical withdrawal symptoms very similar to anxiety, but since they're controllable with alcohol, chances are you won't see a full-blown panic attack; it's true that the suicide rate is 50 times higher for those with alcohol dependence than the general population, but any previous depression they suffer is often well-masked by the drink; although when things are really bad they may hallucinate, they clearly don't have the same bizarre thought patterns as someone with schizophrenia; they may suffer intense obsessional jealousy, but everyone has some quirk or other, don't they?

Alcohol dependence is not a dramatic form of breakdown: it's gradual and it fits neatly into the rest of our lives. Unlike heroin addiction or compulsive eating, it's a long time before it needs to have a secret side to it. To use the analogy of the car once more, it's more like finding you have to put more and more oil in to get the car to function properly. You can get away with this for quite a time (depending on the make and history of the car), but eventually you have to acknowledge that your car has a major problem which makes its normal use impossible.

The problems are psychological, social, financial, legal, and physical. The psychological effects include those related to the dependence itself: the feelings of tension, anxiety and irritability that come when you feel you need a drink, as well as the depression as one part of you acknowledges that things are getting out of control. They also involve the personality changes that occur as people become increasingly loquacious, boastful, offensive and boring. Recent research has shown that male drinkers especially are less able to judge people's expressions of disgust and anger, and so they will be without the feedback that the rest of us use to help maintain our social skills.

As a heavy drinker you may find yourself suffering memory blackouts and being dependent on alcohol often involves increasingly poor memory. Geoff Lowe, from the University of Hull, has shown that things learnt while under the influence of alcohol are more easily forgotten when sober, but can be remembered again when drinking recommences. This 'state-dependent' learning may have some implications in encouraging you to continue drinking, but also causes obvious problems in a marriage where the Jekyll-and-Hyde phenomenon of living with a heavy drinker is exacerbated even more by the fact that you can't remember conversations that occurred in the sober or the drunk state when you're in the other state.

The social part of the breakdown is the risk that you place on your marriage and other relationships, and on your place in society. While alcohol appears to be a large factor in the number of women divorcing their husbands, it is even larger when men divorcing their wives are studied. This probably reflects society's attitude of greater tolerance towards drunken men than drunken women. The financial consequences can be assessed by keeping an accurate diary of what you drink in a week (see p. 147). However, they also come from losing jobs and becoming gradually more unable to find new ones. The men and women slumped in doorways at Kings Cross Station, or its equivalent in any city of the world, all started life with the usual variety of aspirations and occupations. They include lawyers and directors alongside labourers and messengers: addiction certainly has no class barriers. The legal part is the enormously increased chance that you will be charged with drunken driving, assaults both inside and outside the home, child abuse and even murder. In a study which looked at family violence and alcohol, more than half of the 'battered wives' studied reported partners who were heavy drinkers. There are often links with other addictive behaviours such as drug abuse and gambling, and criminal activity may be involved in supporting an addiction.

There is not a single cell in the body that is unaffected by alcohol. More specifically, the physical breakdown shows itself in liver damage such as cirrhosis (a particularly unpleasant way to die) which continues to climb all over the world in direct proportion to alcohol consumption. Certainly in men, though less so in women, the damage can actually be mended in its early stages by stopping drinking. It also increases the chances of breast cancer in women and cancer of the oesophagus, throat and mouth, and ulcers of the stomach and duodenum in both sexes. While it is clear that alcohol can have a bad effect upon heart muscle and is associated with a greater likelihood of having strokes, there is still no conclusive evidence to support the claim that moderate drinking actually *reduces* heart conditions.

Prolonged alcohol abuse may also lead to brain damage: general intellectual functioning is impaired and brain scans reveal that brain tissue is lost, but some at least is regained with abstinence. The worst effects on the brain are seen in Korsakoff's syndrome which is a form of dementia and incurable. I remember Eddie, once a company director, ambling along the corridors of the hospital where I worked, showing people his label which told him which ward he now called home. He would be directed, but within 30 seconds would have forgotten and have to ask all over again. Women are more susceptible than men to the effects of alcohol, especially in terms of liver damage.

Less well known but equally devastating are the effects on your sex life. With prolonged heavy drinking men may lose their sex drive and, as their penises, testes and sperm count shrivel away, they also become impotent and sterile. With very high alcohol consumption a large proportion of men lose body hair and develop breasts. The opposite effects occur for women who may also suffer menstrual difficulties. Heavy drinking during pregnancy creates great risks to the unborn child, and little or no alcohol is usually the safest rule at that time.

These features of alcohol abuse come together to provide us with short-hand tests to decide whether or not our drinking is out of hand. There are a number of more sophisticated assessments, but a simple one uses the categories of problems provided by Roizen, an American sociologist, and called the '4 Ls': if your liver, your lover (partners, family or friends), your livelihood, or your dealings with the law have been affected by repeated alcohol use, then you should recognise that it's likely you have a problem. A more scientific test of alcohol dependence asks you the following questions:

Circle correct answer

1 Do you feel you are a normal drinker?   YES NO

2 Do friends or relatives think you are a normal   YES NO
   drinker?

3 Have you ever attended a meeting of   YES NO
   Alcoholics Anonymous?

4 Have you ever lost friends or girlfriends or   YES NO
   boyfriends because of drinking?

5 Have you ever got into trouble at work   YES NO
   because of drinking?

6 Have you ever neglected your obligations,   YES NO
   your family, or your work for two or more days
   in a row because you were drinking?

7 Have you ever had delirium tremors (DTs),   YES NO
   severe shaking, heard voices or seen things
   that were not there after heavy drinking?

8 Have you ever gone to anyone for help about   YES NO
   your drinking?

9 Have you ever been in a hospital because of   YES NO
   drinking?

10 Have you ever been arrested for drunken   YES NO
   driving or driving after drinking?

An answer 'no' to questions 1 and 2 and an answer 'yes' to questions 4, 5, 6, and 10 yields two points each; and an answer 'yes' to 3, 7, 8 and 9 yields five points each. A total score of 5 points or more is taken as a diagnosis of alcohol dependence.*

* From Pokomy, A.D. et al., (1972). *American Journal of Psychiatry*, *129*, 342–345.

Despite such useful indicators, many people still refuse to acknowledge that they have a problem, even when their marriage has ended, their driving licence has been taken away, their job is under threat, their finances are often problematic, their friends are reduced to a number of other 'hard' drinkers, they've had warnings about their liver, and so on.

Mick, a journalist on a national paper, had suffered all these setbacks, apart from job-loss. Like most newspaper offices, his was remarkably tolerant of alcohol use both on and off the premises, and so he was able to see his drinking as normal within the context in which he worked. He would point particularly to others who 'just liked a drink and a good time' and remained able to ignore the fact that these were people with equal problems, most of whom had themselves suffered psychological and social consequences of dependence. Like most problem drinkers, he blamed external causes for his difficulties: his wife had ended the marriage because of her intolerance and lack of fun; another driver had caused the accident that got him banned; his doctor was just plain mistaken in his interpretation of his liver function tests. His denial reminded one of the poor, spotty youth in the anti-heroin campaign who continued to say to the end, 'I can handle it.' You *must* accept fully that you've got a problem and that it's *your* problem, not anyone else's, before change is possible.

WHAT CAUSES IT?

Given such a dreadful list of the consequences of alcohol dependence, what on earth makes someone continue in a behaviour which destroys both the individual and those around him or her? Well, the most clear-cut factor is of course the alcohol itself. Some people consider that if you drink enough of it for long enough eventually you are bound to become dependent: it's the regular drinking that causes dependence, while occasional bout-drinking causes accidents and social harm. How little you should drink to avoid these problems is the subject of constant research. Damage to your health becomes likely once you're drinking more than 35 units a week (21 for a woman), and the Royal College of Psychiatrists' latest book, *Alcohol: Our Favourite Drug*, says that damage will increase *greatly* after 50 units of alcohol a week (an average of about 3½ pints of beer a day) for men, or 35 for women. Anyone who wants to drink regularly should therefore aim well below these levels. The number of units in pub measures of drinks are as follows:

1 Unit	=	½ pint of ordinary beer of lager	=	*A single measure of spirits (whisky, gin, bacardi, vodka etc)	=	A glass of wine	=	A small glass of sherry	=	A measure of Vermouth or Aperitif

The Health Education Council suggests that you are unlikely to be damaging yourself if you drink less than 22 units per week (11 pints of beer) as a man and less than 15 as a woman.

Unlike many other forms of psychological behaviour, alcohol use and abuse is one which has woven in and out of the criminal law, and its illegality or not has often depended on whether alcohol dependence was seen as a disease or a habit. Certainly the disease model of 'the alcoholic' who suffered from 'alcoholism' did much to increase tolerance towards those who were dependent, but, like all illness models of psychological problems, it tends to relieve the individual of the responsibility for change. This of course isn't an inevitable result of an illness model but for people who are already giving causes outside themselves for their problems, it's certainly a risk.

The idea that alcohol dependence is a disease is the basis of organisations like Alcoholics Anonymous and has a clear advantage for some problem drinkers in that it gives them no alternative but to stop drinking completely. There have been various mechanisms proposed for the way the disease might operate: it may be in the form of an allergy to alcohol, or there may be physiological factors which make the effects more potent or dependence more likely. These theories all have problems and none quite fit the facts (see Heather and Robertson's book for a critique) but certainly there is some genetic evidence which suggests that severe alcohol

* This applies to the ⅙ gill measure used in most of England and Wales. But in some places, pub measures are larger than this. In Northern Ireland a pub measure is ¼ gill. In Scotland it can be either ⅕ gill or ¼ gill.

problems may be inherited, at least in males. This research largely used adoption studies, and so ruled out some of the chance that there was an environmental cause to the dependence, though recently these types of studies have had major criticisms from parts of the scientific world. Obviously in cases where children are growing up with a problem drinker, they are going to be affected in some way, and modelling themselves on their parent is sadly frequent, perhaps partly as a way of saying 'Look what you've done to me.' Those in high-risk jobs, such as seamen or publicans or journalists, are pointed to as arguments for the environmental lobby; but it's equally possible that people enter such a job because they are attracted (by reason of their physical make-up) to the free and easy lifestyle.

Psychoanalytic theories of alcohol dependence are based around the notion that alcohol provides an escape from reality. One proposes that, because of very early problems in the parent–child relationship, the person becomes 'fixed' to some extent at the very earliest, 'oral' stage of development and so shows the characteristics of needing comfort by the mouth, being very dependent and having little self-control. A theory which has more use in actually providing help, is one that sees alcohol consumption as essentially a self-destructive behaviour resulting from repressed anger and frustration at a parent's early behaviour towards the child. Maggie described how well this seemed to fit her case:

My father was killed in the war just a few weeks after I was born. My mother was forced to work in a factory and I was apparently left in the charge of various neighbours and my older brother, when he was not at school. Presumably this left much to be desired in terms of having a loving early childhood. In fact my mother worked all my life. She had to in order to keep us. I loved her enormously and when she died I was completely demolished for weeks. I was 19 then, and I began to drink to help with the grief I felt. And it worked too. I stayed a heavy drinker all through my student days, but eased off a bit in the first few years of my marriage. Then, when my husband started having affairs, it all began again, only more so, and when he finally left me I really went to town.

Thanks to my friends, I eventually got help from a variety of sources. One was a Gestalt therapist who made me look at last at my anger over my childhood. It was at first impossibly hard to acknowledge: my mother had done everything she could for me, so how could I be angry?

How could anyone be angry with someone they loved? It was only when I finally got in touch with all the hurt and rage I'd felt, that I was able to start really wanting to stop drinking. Her explanation was that I'd been turning all that against myself, rather than my mother, and used the booze both to hide from the reality and to harm myself for deep down daring to be angry with someone I loved so much, especially as her death made any expression of this conflict to her no longer possible. When my husband betrayed me it again woke up these early feelings. It made a lot of sense to me, all that.

A criticism of this theory of self-destruction is that it doesn't explain why someone should turn to alcohol rather than any other means, but this seems irrelevant: presumably you turn to the drug that gives you the best results. For some people this may well be heroin or cocaine, but for far more it will be alcohol, simply because it's so much more easily obtainable and acceptable. Others may simply experience their conflict as depression. There are certainly many reasons why we do choose alcohol, and these form the basis of the behavioural theories that alcohol dependence is learnt.

Like all addictions – gambling, compulsive eating, heroin, whatever – people learn to use alcohol because it provides them with something better than not using it. In Maggie's case it gave her relief from her grief and feelings she found unacceptable; for others it may make social situations less frightening, alter a lack of confidence, make them feel less lonely, or become 'one of the boys' – or nowadays 'one of the girls'. In our society, it can appear almost impossible to have a social life which does not include the use of alcohol. As dependence grows, it also gives relief from the physical symptoms of withdrawal. So built into yourself or built into your environment are numerous factors which make alcohol rewarding, just as there may equally be factors which make it the opposite – a determination not to be like your father, a religious conversion, a strong sense of your own worth, and so on. As Heather and Robertson point out, there are as many reasons why someone should or should not become a problem drinker as there are individuals. But that doesn't mean it's impossible to find the factors that prompt the drinking and deal with them.

TREATMENT

On the whole the use of alcohol wards in mental hospitals is not particularly common in Britain, though in the States, where it's still largely seen as a disease, such units are still regularly used. It makes little sense to take people out of the environment which, at least partly if not wholly, prompted them to drink; to dry them out and then to send them back to the same lethal environment, and expect to have solved their problems. However, it may clearly be necessary, if someone is physically very debilitated through alcohol abuse or if they have no fixed social structure to support them, to hospitalise them till their physical symptoms are over and till they are clear where they will be living and what supports will be available.

Drug treatment is rarely used, though occasionally psychiatrists will give some medication to those who are alcohol (or heroin) dependent in order to relieve the more severe withdrawal symptoms; others will refuse to substitute one drug for another in this way. The drug which is most commonly associated with alcohol dependence is Antabuse which when taken regularly makes the person extremely nauseated should she or he drink any alcohol. Because this puts responsibility outside of the drinker, it's not a very useful long-term strategy. Ideally it should not be used except as a stop-gap while drinkers begin to get their lives in order.

Alcoholics Anonymous has been operating for over 50 years and its methods of group support for total abstinence and progression through a series of steps have helped millions. It's impossible to say whether one approach to alcoholism or problem drinking is much better than another, since most people stop drinking fairly easily for a time, but then begin again with all the same intensity. I am aware of some alcohol services which count the mere stopping as a success, whereas we can only look at long-term abstinence or control as bringing about the sort of change that matters.

Once they reach the difficult point of realising they have a problem, very few heavy drinkers decide that they need abstinence; most begin by approaching their difficulties with some form of controlled drinking, or by using local NHS services. There's no doubt that some of these will have success. Of those who don't manage to control their lives in this way, a number will join AA and begin to work their way through the programme they offer.

The actor Antony Hopkins is one who has described this process and the enormous benefits the organization has brought him. It's certainly true that the changes I've seen in alcoholics' lives (as well as those of their families) which AA has brought about are by no means superficial or limited just to abstinence, but very much more akin to the process that you experience with some forms of psychotherapy.

ACCEPT is a more recently formed organisation which agrees there may be alternatives to abstinence, though in practice finds that most of its clients learn they must abstain for the rest of their lives. Unlike Alcoholics Anonymous, they do not see the problem as a disease, but as a symptom that something is wrong in a person's life.

One of the main arguments against the disease model of 'alcoholism' and insistence that abstinence is the only cure comes from the fact that many of you who are alcohol dependent (or addicted to any other drug or behaviour) manage to cut down to acceptable levels by yourselves when some aspect of your life changes. You may marry or have a child and decide perhaps that you want a different family life from your own; you may join a religion where alcohol is not acceptable except in small amounts; you may get a marvellous job where driving is essential; or you may lose the job and simply have no money to support the addiction. For some of you such life changes may be as effective as any form of counselling.

It is this ability for people to change their own lives in some way which lets them control their drinking that forms part of the rationale for a behavioural approach to therapy. This teaches you to change aspects of your environment or your skills in order to unlearn the alcohol-dependent behaviours you've learned over the years.

Clive was referred by his general practitioner to a clinical psychologist. He was overweight and unhealthy; his liver function test had sounded warning bells; and his marriage was precarious. He was very behind with his work, and clearly depressed. He was asked to spend the next two weeks keeping a diary about how much and what he drank and when, what the circumstances were, in whose company, and so on. A page of this is shown opposite. When people keep diaries to investigate a behaviour they invariably cut down on it considerably (see p. 134) and Clive considered he'd not had an abnormally large amount, apart from on

Day	What did you drink?	When/Where/Who with? (add any event which seemed to trigger the drinking.)	Units	Total
Monday	2 pints beer	Lunchtime in pub with colleagues	4	
	2½ pints beer	After work in pub with colleagues	5	
	1 can Special Brew	Watching 9 o'clock news, alone	4	13
Tuesday	1 pint of beer	Lunchtime in pub with colleagues	2	
	3 large whiskies	Spread over evening, either with wife or alone	6	8
Wednesday	2 pints beer	Lunchtime in pub with colleagues	4	
	4 glasses wine	With wife over dinner (bought on the way home)	4	
	1 large whisky	Nightcap	2	10
Thursday	1 pint beer	After work in pub alone	2	
	⅓ bottle of whisky	Working on report till early hours – alone but after argument with wife about how much I drank – I'd had so little today	10	12
Friday	2 large whiskies	Early lunch, feeling fragile – in pub alone	4	
	3 pints beer	After work in pub with colleagues	6	10
Saturday	2 cans Special Brew	During afternoon, wife was anxious about the dinner we were giving, I felt anxious too, as a result	8	
	2 gin and tonics	Dinner party with wife and friends, feeling anxious		
	1 bottle wine		18	
	2 large whiskies	knowing wife was getting angry		26
Sunday	2 pints beer	Took kids to playground at pub – lunchtime	4	
	2 cans Special Brew	Evening, watching TV	8	12
TOTAL FOR WEEK				91

Saturday. He was surprised to find he was drinking a dangerously high number of units. It provided him too with a clear reason why he would be behind with his work: he was hungover all morning and inebriated most of the afternoon! He was then asked to drink nothing for three weeks and to keep a diary about when he felt like drinking; how strong was the urge; and in which situations he gave in.

I actually found I had very little trouble abstaining. Again, this surprised me a lot. I had shaky hands in the morning, but nothing unbearable. In some ways I really enjoyed the challenge. At the same time there were clear periods when I wanted to drink, and I could see from the diary that these came mainly from interactions with people. If I had an argument with my wife I always longed to go and empty a bottle of whisky. When I really thought about this, the feeling behind it seemed to be 'that will show her' – a punishment or something! What was fascinating was that the same sort of feeling came on me when I didn't get enough praise from my boss. My therapist suggested maybe that praise had not been something too free-flowing in my childhood, and he was certainly right there. If I came second in my class, they always wanted to know why!

Clive changed his drinking pattern so that he never drank at lunchtime, but substituted a walk round a gallery or bookshop, or the park, or a lunchtime concert: it's no good cutting out a behaviour you've done for a long time without finding a pleasant and rewarding one to put in its place. Through role play he learnt how to say no to the after-work swill, and began walking home instead of catching the bus. He was quite promptly rewarded by weight loss and admiration, and not only by his wife. He was enjoying his work much more and doing it well now, and he was taught to change his self-talk so that he could praise himself rather than always hoping someone else would. At the same time, he asked his boss to give him more feedback, both positive and negative. Clive found, with the help of relaxation training, that he was able to have a glass of wine with his wife and to save the rest for tomorrow: he seemed to have learned to control his drinking.

Nevertheless, when things went wrong he still found himself going through a few days of alcohol abuse which left him guilty and wretched. During one of these bouts he went to an AA meeting (where, incidentally, he found his GP was a member) and decided that it was easier to give in finally to acknowledging that he was still damaging his life and that abstinence didn't mean he wasn't a real man. He stopped drinking from that day.

'It's funny, you know,' he said after three months of his new life. 'I used to think I was drinking because I was depressed, but now I really think it was the drinking that actually made me depressed.'

There is a wide variety of methods used in behaviour therapy which involve both changing aspects of your environment, changing the way you think about yourself and react to others, and learning new skills. Each person will require different aspects; for example, you may need to be taught assertiveness training and social skills to help you mix socially without the crutch of alcohol; or relaxation as a way to cope with the tension that previously brought on an urge to drink. If you find that feeling low is a cue for you to drink you may need to make a list of substitute enjoyable activities that provide you with pleasure.

Most people who are problem drinkers try at some stage to stop drinking or to control it better. Some of you will be successful and some will not: it usually won't work unless you change something in your life, and a book such as *Let's Drink to Your Health* may provide all the self-help mechanisms you need. One step up from this would be the group called Drinkwatchers, akin to Weight Watchers, (which is a self-help organisation and an offshoot of ACCEPT that teaches ways of drinking less dangerously). An organisation like ACCEPT will, with the aid of your doctor, help you to choose whether abstinence is the way for you, or whether you need psychological or counselling help to work out a successful strategy of controlled drinking. If you feel abstinence is the only way you can also approach Alcoholics Anonymous. Alternatively your GP may refer you to local NHS addiction services.

HELP FOR THE RELATIVES

Being married to someone who is a problem drinker, whether dependent or not, is never easy. When Dylan Thomas wrote *Under Milk Wood* and had Mrs Cherry Owen so tolerant and agreeable to her constantly inebriated husband, his writing was far more likely to be Thomas's own wish-fulfilment than his actual experience. It's true that some children will defend themselves against the disappointment and humiliation by concentrating on the comical side of a drunken parent. George Bernard Shaw, for example, gave this account of the way he and the family treated his father's alcoholism:

> *Drunk or sober, he was usually amiable; but the drunkenness was so humiliating that it would have been unendurable if we had not taken refuge in laughter. It had to be either a family tragedy or a family joke; and it was on the whole a healthy instinct that decided us to get what ribald fun was possible out of it, which however was very little indeed . . .*

On the whole problem drinkers are rarely amusing to those who have to see them often, and the ordinary things for which members of a family come to depend upon each other gradually disappear: finances and good judgement fade away, appointments and birthdays are forgotten, and so on. The constant disappointment that these family members face when their hopes for something different are so regularly dashed can make the children very wary of their own judgement. And, of course, most domestic violence is related to alcohol abuse and many children suffer not only humiliation but also physical and sexual abuse at the hands of an alcoholic parent.

Whether a parent becomes either a buffoon or a beast when he or she is drinking, research shows that a large proportion of their children are affected, showing more signs of anxiety and depression and disturbed behaviour at school than those with sober parents. Paul was 11 when he was sent to an assessment centre to look into his aggressive behaviour to other children. His father was a very heavy drinker and often violent towards his mother during the rows they had over alcohol and their lack of finances. Paul would sometimes try to break up these rows: when he was young he would try to make them laugh, but now he was older he had tried on two occasions to beat off his father. For this he was humiliated – his father holding him by his hair at arm's length to emphasise his small size, and banging him around the head. He obviously found it impossible to understand how his mother would later 'forgive and forget' his father's violence until the next time.

Apart from help for Paul, the social worker involved also provided support for the mother to help her to separate from her husband (who still saw the problem as Paul's) and then encouraged her to join AlAnon while Paul joined AlAteen, the offshoots of Alcoholics Anonymous formed to help relatives and children of those who are dependent on alcohol. If you are in this position, either as a son or daughter, or as a spouse, these organisations will provide important support. Chances are you often feel helpless and almost guilty that nothing that you do can help the person you're attached to and quite possibly still love. These groups will help you to stop seeing yourself as a failure and hopefully will get you to accept that the person's dependency is not your responsibility but his or her own; that it can never be cured by you but only by the relative accepting that there is a problem and deciding for him or herself to do something about it.

In her book, *Women Who Love Too Much*, Robin Norwood puts forward her view that a large number of women become involved with men who are inadequate in some way (alcoholic, addicted to drugs or gambling, violent, or weighed down by their own personality problems) in order to unconsciously try to rectify something that's gone wrong in their early relationships. They may do this over and over again, thinking that this time they will be able to make things right. Theresa married two men both dependent on alcohol. She described to me her first meetings with each of them:

Tom was about ten years older than me. He was a mature student and he'd called round to my room very late one night, pretty drunk. I didn't want the landlady to see him, so I took him out for coffee – thought I'd sober him up. He told me about his dreadful father and how his last wife had been so awful to him, and how he never saw his little girl any more, how he had joined AA, but never went to meetings any more – and so on. By the end of the long tale of woe I was hooked – determined to make it up to him and cure him of his understandable problem.

After a brief tempestuous marriage I managed to get out and my parents and friends sighed with relief – I at least had some sense of self-preservation still. I think I knew that if I stayed I'd have gone under with him, and anyway he was unbearably cruel as well. But did I go and seek a nice steady bloke who hadn't had a ghastly childhood and an ugly past? Did I hell. When I met Charlie he had recently come out of a mental hospital where he'd been drying out. We spent the afternoon drinking by the lake while he told me about his father dying so tragically, his older sister who'd seduced him often, and his dropping out of law school just before he qualified. It was enough. Again I felt myself totally taken over, just like a drug. I can make it right for him I thought. And I spent the next 15 years trying, always unsuccessfully. He was really lovable, not like Tom, but we were hopeless for each other: curing him was accepted by both of us as my responsibility completely, never his. It was my fault I let it go on so long. He was addicted to booze, and I was addicted to trying to control his problem.

Robin Norwood does regard these women as actually 'addicted' to such men, and shows how their behaviour of co-dependency is very similar to other addicts in many respects. She does not see a 'cure' without the help of a support group to keep the sufferer away from her man's problem (or her man); to demonstrate to her how controlling her behaviour actually is; and to explore what went wrong in her own family that she is still trying to make things right: the more hopeless the case the better she'll like it! While she only talks about women in this way, I have met a number (albeit much smaller) of men who similarly go around picking up and helping equally unrewarding women. The book shows you how to start your own self-help group for this, and a number have started since its publication, but AlAnon Family Groups will also provide support in this area.

OTHER ADDICTIONS

As I said at the beginning of the chapter, whatever your addiction you will recognise a number of aspects of alcohol dependency which apply to you. As a relative or friend you are likely to suffer in ways not so unlike those described above. There a number of associations described in the Appendix which will put you on the right track, or ask your doctor, local information office, or Citizens Advice Bureau for information on local agencies.

Chapter

11

Psychological problems in children and adolescents

Children suffer from many of the same psychological problems as adults, often just briefly as part of a developmental stage. The signs that these are occurring are sometimes different to those in adults, and may take a variety of forms. Because of this, we may miss them and as parents find ourselves and our child on the wrong path altogether.

Charlotte at last reached the consultant paediatrician for her tummy aches. Her parents were convinced there was something physically wrong with her, and had insisted on a second opinion. She was a very intelligent and pretty little girl of seven, but she did look a bit washed out and tired. Her mother sat close beside her and put her arm round her daughter to give her an affectionate squeeze and an encouraging smile. Her father just looked worried.

After a thorough physical examination in which she found nothing abnormal, the consultant asked more detailed questions about the family. Charlotte was an only child; her mum was an actress, but had stopped working until Charlotte was old enough to go to school. It was difficult trying to get back after such a break but it wouldn't have been right, she said, to be absent when her daughter was so young. Now she had to grab every opportunity she could. The father was a journalist, and had been able to stagger his hours so he was always there when Charlotte came home from school. Charlotte's tummy aches had started about a year ago and came on most violently first thing in the morning and usually subsided by lunchtime. Sometimes they would happen in the night and then she would swop places with dad and sleep with mum. Rubbing her tummy gently eased the pain a little bit.

'Our GP obviously thought it was all put on to stop going to school,' said the mother, 'But she does very well at school, and she'd certainly looked forward to going there. She couldn't wait. It might be hard for you to believe, but her pain is very real. She's doubled up with it sometimes.'

The consultant assured the mother that she didn't doubt for one moment that Charlotte's tummy aches were real, but that, since there wasn't a physical cause for them, maybe Charlotte was worrying about something?

'Well, I suppose it could be the school. We live in a rather working-class area and so there's not all that many middle-class kids in the school. She's never said she gets bullied or anything like that, but I can imagine she might feel a bit of an outsider sometimes. I have actually been to talk to the teachers but they say Charlotte has plenty of friends there. Still, they can't see everything, can they?'

The psychologist in the team offered to have a chat to see if he could find out if this was true. The teachers at the school assured him that there was actually quite a large number of children there just as bright as Charlotte, and that when she did come to school she quickly settled and played well with the other children. So it was time to think about the family itself. There was no doubt that Charlotte was well loved and looked after: not many mothers would have given up such a budding career for six years. That must be quite a responsibility for a child to shoulder. Perhaps that was one clue. The other was the complete absence of any acknowledgement that Charlotte might be upset by her mother's absences. They were obviously very close, and it couldn't be easy for her.

Her mother became very defensive about this, but was persuaded that it wasn't that her absences were wrong, but they were being treated as if they didn't matter. She agreed to try things out for a few months: firstly, not to mention again the difficulties caused by the break in her career (it was after all her decision, not Charlotte's); and secondly, to openly talk to her daughter about what it must feel like whenever she left. In other words, she was giving Charlotte permission to feel sad, rather than swallowing it up into her tummy and making it feel so sore. Like many interventions with children, this worked a treat and the child's stomach aches had gone completely within a couple of months.

There seem to be two reasons why we, as parents, so often miss a child's unhappiness or anxiety. First, it's not easy for children to actually know that they're sad or tense, so they often won't be able to tell you: it's usually up to you to raise the possibility with them. The second reason is that we don't really want to know. If our child is unhappy we instantly assume that it's our fault and that we've done something wrong. It is hard for us as parents to accept that all parents make mistakes – lots of them – and many of us are forced, like Charlotte's mother, to make compromises in the way we bring up our children. It's pretending the mistake or compromise hasn't happened that causes the real problems. This shifts the onus onto the child: they are 'ill' in some way, or they are 'terribly badly behaved'.

This refusal to acknowledge that children do get hurt by us and by the events that they experience goes right through society; for example with the adage, 'Children are resilient'. Such a myth not only allows 'good enough' parents to ignore their mistakes, but also permits bad parents to take out their frustrations on their children, as if they were made of something as resilient as a punchbag. You still hear fathers (in particular) say: 'Well, a good beating never did me any harm' – ignoring the fact that, at the very least, it probably helped to turn them into child beaters.

Although young people suffer from adult disorders too, the proviso from the introduction that there are no really clear-cut categories of psychological problems applies even more strongly to them. Feeling scared or feeling sad can appear in all sorts of ways in children: by physical problems, by bed-wetting, soiling, behaviour problems, obsessions, phobias, by becoming mute, as well as by clear-cut depression and anxiety. For this reason I'm joining together a number of problems under the general heading of 'anxiety and depression'. More specific problems will be discussed at the end of the chapter.

ANXIETY AND DEPRESSION

Before the age of two, children's needs for food, comfort, love, warmth, security and stimulation are hopefully met to a large extent by a parent-figure. These needs are never met perfectly because we have to learn to 'read' our infants – to know when a cry means hunger and when it means 'I want a cuddle' – and also because none of us are perfect parents. Infants' needs are immediate – you can't distract them for long, as any parent knows. Of course, in some children these needs will not be met. I don't just mean the extreme cases that fill our newspapers, of torture and starvation; but rather the type of case where a parent-figure is constantly depressed and cannot face playing with the child, or where a mother meets her own unmet needs for love and security with something to eat, and so in turn provides only food for her child, irrespective of why it's crying. But these cases are the rare ones; generally speaking our babies get roughly what they need.

Around the age of two, the parent-figure changes a little. Instead of providing just what a child wants when it wants it, he or she begins to put demands on the child: wait until lunchtime for your food; use the potty instead of your knickers; don't touch mummy's breasts; don't murder your new sister; and so on. The child learns that, although it wants to carry on as before, the parent demands that it change its behaviour to something more socially acceptable. The conflict this causes produces the raging tantrums of the terrible two's. As the child reaches school age, it gradually learns to 'internalise' these external demands, to be able to provide them for himself or herself, and so develops a conscience. This produces just the same conflicts, but the battles go on more inside than out, and the conflict produces anxiety, a fear that something dangerous might happen: mummy won't love me as much if I do that, for example. We have to confront anxieties all our lives, and most of us learn to cope with them, one way or another. But often, even in the best of homes, children face situations of conflict which they find threatening and which they've not yet learnt to successfully overcome. How they react may take as many forms as there are children!

Mark's father had left home when he was four. His mother was very upset and cried quite a lot. Mark began wetting the bed again and sleeping badly. He was very clingy to his mother and seemed to be frightened that she too would leave him. This general state of anxiety developed gradually into a phobia that a murderer would come and kill his mother and his father. Although he could be reassured about his mother by checking the locks of the house with her, he would sometimes get in such a state about his father, that his mother would phone him and get him to come over. So, in a sad way both Mark and his mother were being rewarded by his phobia.

By watching him play with dolls representing his family, his therapist quickly realised that Mark was very angry with his father for leaving (but had to put his anger out onto a murderer), and also with his mother because she 'must have done something to make him go away'. This was actually safer for him than to acknowledge the underlying anxiety that *he* had somehow driven his father away. If he showed his anger to her, he thought she might go away too. Children of Mark's age often think they're much more powerful than they are, and so they secretly fear they cause everything that goes wrong.

Simon's parents were both teachers. He'd always done well at school himself, but not without some effort. They took it for granted that he'd get his 'A' levels and go on to university. At 15 he switched friends abruptly and began to mix with a gang who'd left school the year before. They professed themselves to be anarchists, and dressed in a way to make any parent appalled. Although Simon continued at school, he did no further work, claiming school was an institution of the state, and so failed all his exams and left. To his parents he was constantly aggressive and abusive, sneering at their capitalist lifestyle, calling them hypocrites, and so on. A good friend of theirs, who'd watched it all from the wings, suggested to Simon that it must have been really hard having to live up to such high expectations. Simon agreed it certainly was, and admitted to feeling pretty anxious about it for a couple of years. And maybe it had felt safer to opt out of school than to sit the exams and fail? Simon admitted that was true. In his eyes the political stance had given him a cover that allowed him to still relate to his parents, albeit belligerently: if he'd failed he thought they'd give him up for ever.

Children may experience anxiety in much the same way as adults (see Chapters 3 and 4). It may stay as a collection of anxiety symptoms without a focus or, more usually, may develop into something more specific; for example, Mark's murderer who symbolised his own anger, or a child who develops obsessional problems. It's worth knowing that children can also experience full-blown panic attacks just as frightening as any adult. These may, for example, occur in adolescents as they experience their first sexual longings but find them terrifying because of the guilt and shame they produce.

Another way children express their anxiety is by school phobia or, more accurately, school refusal. Their constant absence from school is seen as due either to obvious anxiety at the thought of it, or to physical symptoms such as stomach pains, headaches, or sore joints. Occasionally the school will really be the source of the problem but, more often, it involves some sort of fear about being separated from a parent. Although Charlotte was showing one form of this, most seem to develop from the child's not wanting to leave a parent home alone. When the relationship is explored, it's often the case that the parent doesn't actually *want* to be left home alone, and so the child is really just doing what the parent wants: for example, where a father has died or left the family home, and the child and mother provide support for each other. Parents should try to make the initial effort of getting their son or daughter to school, hopefully with help from an outside therapist, and then they can look at what emerges in themselves when the child is no longer at home all day.

Many children suffer from bedwetting (eneuresis) during periods of stress, and if it only lasts a few weeks, there's nothing to worry about. However, around a tenth of children, especially boys, have still not become dry by the time they start school and others will become wet again around that time. If this persists, then help should be sought, first of all by approaching your doctor. If a child has never been dry, day or night, then it may be that the bladder has a smaller capacity than the average and needs training in order to stretch it a little. Or, with bedwetting, it may be that he's a particularly heavy sleeper, or simply has a nervous system that's maturing more slowly than usual. Emotional distress in the first place is only one of the possible causes. But even where bedwetting is handled well by parents – without blame, with the minimum of fuss, and certainly never with punishment – it can still lead to future distress from the smell that is difficult to control, from the impossibility of going to sleep with friends, or going camping, and so on. There are a number of methods to cure the problem, and your doctor will either be able to help you with these or refer you to a psychologist.

Children have usually learnt bowel control – both when to go and when not to go – by the time they're three, and if there is still a problem in this area by the time they're four, then help should be sought. Children may soil themselves occasionally as a reaction to severe emotional distress. This may be just an isolated event (comparable to adults having diarrhoea when faced with something very stressful), or may be part of some general 'going back to babyhood', or regression; for example, they may want a bottle, or suck their thumbs, or return to baby talk. It's their way of showing that at that time they need the security and comfort of being a baby. Being given a little dose of this may quickly cure the problem, but if it persists, then help should be sought.

Soiling is sometimes also the only way children have of showing parents they're angry with them. In this case these otherwise well-behaved children will either soil or hold onto their faeces like grim death! This may happen where a parent, usually the mother, is particularly controlling of the child's life, and very over-protective or a perfectionist. The child will often have been potty-trained very young, even by the age of one, and there may be a very close relationship between the child and the mother, with the father rather distant from them both.

It's important to realise that, like all the other behaviours or symptoms that are the result of some anxiety, the child is completely unaware of what's actually behind the problem. For this reason, both the child and the parents may be happy to see it as physical. Certainly, retention of faeces can occasionally be physical, due to a very sore area inside the anus, but this can easily be recognised. After it has been ruled out, it's important to seek psychological help. Apart from relieving the child of its problems, it will often let the parents recognise, and so relieve, their own distress.

Children often go through an obsessional stage, especially when they're young: teddy has to be put on the right of the pillow, never on the left; the counterpane must always be a certain way; the door must be left three inches ajar, no more and no less, and so on. These stages only last a few months, and are nothing to worry about. Obsessions which appear later and which continue for a long time may signal more severe anxiety and help should be sought for this, especially if the behaviours are being added to and it's clear the child is unable to stop them. They may involve the types of behaviour described in Chapter 8, or they may involve a whole series of internal rituals which the child needs to go through to ward off the obsessional thoughts. At such times, the child will appear very distracted and withdrawn. Sometimes parents may find themselves drawn into the rituals – *they* have to do X, Y or Z so the child can relax. Like all obsessional disorders, catching the problem early is an important key to successful change.

Depression is often another product of anxiety, or it may exist on its own; there's still considerable confusion about diagnosing depression in children and adolescents because, like anxiety, it appears in so many ways. However, occasionally there is no doubt that a child is depressed: the weeping, the loss of interest in activities, and the difficulty in concentrating tell us as clearly as they do in adults. Other ways of letting us know something is definitely wrong include self-mutilation (for example, cutting at themselves), running away, and suicide attempts, whether or not they were meant to fail. Far more commonly, children express their unhappiness through physical symptoms, by behaving badly or by withdrawing. The young people below illustrate some of these reactions.

Steve was 10 when his younger brother died from head injuries after a horse-riding accident. Of course, his parents' grief was enormous and, understandably, they could think of little else for quite some time. Steve's own tears took place mainly in his room and, with his parents he would often try to jolly them up in ways hopelessly inappropriate to a mourning household. His father soon buried his grief in work, and his mother began to notice Steve again, especially when he mentioned that he had awful headaches. When these continued she became understandably overprotective of her only child, and took him around a series of doctors who all pronounced him physically well. Most of them suggested a child psychiatrist or psychologist, but she was reluctant to entertain this possibility. Eventually it was an educational psychologist attached to the school who was able to suggest to the parents the link between Steve's headaches and his brother's head injuries; to gently point out that Steve had not really been allowed to grieve with his parents; and, difficult though it might be, to stress the importance that Steve should be loved now for himself, and not because he was all that was left.

Because society (of which we're all members) maintains the reassuring myth that children are resilient, the intensity of their grief when someone close dies or is seriously ill, or leaves, is often overlooked. Perhaps even more so than in adult grief (because adults have learnt more ways of avoiding distressing thoughts), children and adolescents are likely to experience considerable guilt – of course Steve, like any normal child, had thumped his younger brother and felt almost murderous with jealousy at times. This is often mixed with anger at being left with responsibility for keeping the parents happy. And then the anger too just adds to the guilt. At some stage the most useful thing to do is to acknowledge with the child that these feelings often do happen and that it's quite OK to feel angry and to be terribly sad at the same time. Guilt is a harder one to tackle, but sharing your own guilty feelings, and then explaining that they're common but unnecessary, may help a lot. The main thing is to remember that if a child realises that it's OK to have these feelings, they at once become less troublesome and frightening.

Julie was seven when her mother, a pleasant, caring woman, brought her for help. She had seemed so unhappy lately, had spent hours sitting and rocking and moaning, and had talked about sticking a knife into herself. Needless to say, the mother was terribly worried and upset. She explained that ever since her young sister, Rosie, had started at the same school, Julie had become terribly anxious about her school work and also very protective about her sister, worrying all the time that she would be hurt in the playground. Despite the dramatic symptoms, only one consultation was needed. Some simple tests showed Julie that she was just where she should be at school – comfortably average and not behind in any way. It was possible to explain to the mother that Julie was, like all normal children, quite likely to be jealous of her young sister – more so as she'd now taken a position in the school – and she was turning the anger she felt against herself as many children with strong 'consciences' will do. This relieved her mother considerably, especially since she could then recall the murderous rage that *she* had felt towards her own sister when she was young. Julie's over-zealous behaviour in looking after Rosie was probably a protection against her own anger rather than anyone else's!

There was no 'treatment' needed: the mother left resolved to make it clear to Julie how much she valued her in her own right, and how proud she was of her, and to make sure she stopped making any comparisons. Later she wrote saying that the depression seemed to have gone within a couple of days and how Julie seemed happier than she'd done for ages. The sensible woman added how she told Julie (with no mention of Rosie and her), about her own jealousy towards her sister, and how much they later grew to love each other.

Sad or depressed feelings are often a feature of adolescence. It's quite likely that changing hormones play a part in this, but also adolescents are experiencing a multitude of conflicts and anxieties: about changing their height and their shape and so not being sure who they are; about new sexual urges and the feelings of guilt and excitement they bring; about wanting to stay safe in the family, but beginning to need a life of their own. All these mixed emotions also produce some turmoil in the parents, and relationships between them are as rigorously tested as are those between them and their son or daughter. In all this disturbance, relationships can get dreadfully stuck where none of the participants can see below the surface and so the same scenarios are repeated again and again, almost to a script, though all of them long for something different.

Katherine's mother had had a hard time bringing her up single-handed after her husband walked out of their lives. She had remarried when Katherine was 10. Now her daughter was 15 and had only just survived an overdose of paracetamol. The child psychiatrist saw an awkward girl, quite beautiful, but whose movements suggested she was really uncomfortable in her body. She hunched her shoulders and let her hair cover her face. He could see she didn't like herself too much. Her mother had told him of her truancy and rudeness and stealing over the last couple of years. She was pretty sure she'd been experimenting with drugs and she certainly smoked 'secretly' in the house, an activity both her parents abhorred. She had a couple of scars on her arms which her mother described as a 'ridiculous fashion'.

He met with them together and watched Katherine shouting at her mother that she never let her do anything, that she was just old-fashioned and stopped all her pleasure. It was pretty clear to him that in fact the daughter got very little pleasure out of any of her wayward behaviour. He watched the mother furious with Katherine, saying that she was totally selfish and didn't care a jot for anyone but herself; that if she'd only do her exams everything would be O K; that she was totally fed up with the whole house revolving around Katherine. He could see that the mother (and probably everyone else) was seeing her daughter as the only problem in the house, just as she was seeing passing exams as the only solution. It was pretty clear that the mother had suffered herself and needed more support than she was getting. It was clear too that both of them loved each other, but all the words to say it and the actions to show it were buried under the anger. Only when Katherine was drunk would she tell her mother she loved her, and then, of course, it was rarely well received.

Later, during family therapy, it gradually emerged that Katherine had been abused by her real father and he had left when the mother made it clear she knew. At that point it was swept under the carpet, both mother and daughter burying their feelings over what had happened: the daughter's guilt that she had been responsible for her father's leaving and anger that her mother had failed to protect her; and the mother's own guilt and resentment that Katherine's cold angry glare made her feel, which stopped her properly enjoying what she regarded as her last chance of happiness. Perhaps this was why, on the one hand, she was fairly over-protective, and on the other hand, she could ignore the slashed arms as simply fashion. Only when all this could be brought out into the open and the real cause of the feelings could be expressed, were the pair of them able to let each other know about how much they really cared for each other.

This case had more dramatic origins than most, but it's very common for distressed children and adolescents to go through periods of behaviour problems – destroying things, bullying, stealing, constantly being rude and aggravating, and as they get older also drinking, smoking and taking drugs. Depressed adolescents are often particularly and suddenly irritable. As parents we tend to respond to the immediate behaviour; it's certainly not easy, when a child is behaving so abominably, to look beyond this, but it's always worthwhile.

Where problems seem too difficult for simple solutions, a general practitioner may send parents to a child psychologist, child psychiatrist or social worker for help, or the child may be recognised as having difficulties by a teacher or an educational psychologist. As with most childhood disorders, treatments will usually involve behaviour therapy, psychotherapy with the child, help for the parents, or family therapy for everyone. Psychotherapy can be difficult with adolescents because they are at a stage where they are trying to break away from relationships with adults, rather than begin them. However, family therapy is often very useful.

Suicide attempts are becoming more common in adolescents, especially girls, and, although many of them are more cries for help than a real wish to die, an increasing number are of course tragically successful (see p. 78). Even where death was obviously not intended it's very important to make sure that some help and understanding is provided. It's quite understandable that as parents you might be feeling angry: in cases where you feel you're being manipulated, an honest show of anger (as opposed to hostility), may actually be appropriate and 'clear the air'. In other cases, where the child is more clearly depressed, anger is not useful. The risk of actual suicide increases as communication with parents breaks down and so help should be sought to get you talking again – not in the old patterns that have become so hard to change, but in a more useful way. Serious suicide attempts and actual suicides are more common in boys and are a major cause of death in young people. Recently a support group has been formed called Compassionate Friends for parents of young people who have killed themselves.

Drug abuse is not dealt with specifically in this book, though it can clearly be seen as a behaviour disorder and so part of the previous discussion. Probably the majority of adolescents will try marihuana (dope, hash, blow, grass, pot) at some time or another. All the evidence suggests that, taken occasionally, this is a remarkably 'safe' (soft) drug, considerably more so than alcohol or tobacco. Heroin is quite a different thing altogether. Research shows that young people are more likely to take dangerous drugs (heroin and cocaine) if (1) they see themselves as not up-to-the-mark in terms of their friends, and so may deviate in order to gain acceptance; (2) they are strongly influenced by their friends; (3) there is for some reason a weakening of parental or other control; and (4) there is early abuse of alcohol or soft drugs. There are, however, quite a few professional people (some involved in drug rehabilitation) who feel that the severity of the problem of drugs nationally is both a media and a political hype: more sensational but much easier to control than unemployment (which is undoubtedly a factor in young drug abuse). There is, however, no doubt that the numbers of young addicts are increasing, especially amidst the poverty of inner city estates. Addicted young people bring enormous misery to themselves and their families, and nowadays, if they share needles, are prime targets for catching and spreading the AIDS virus. There are a number of good books on the subject, and some of these are listed in the bibliography. Martin Herbert's book, *Living With Teenagers* provides a good overview of normal and problem behaviour in young people.

Other psychological problems of adolescence include eating disorders such as anorexia nervosa (described in detail in Chapter 9), problems with alcohol (Chapter 10), and sex. While young people who have been brought up to regard sex as something rather unpleasant or even downright wicked, are likely to find their sexual urges in adolescence particularly disturbing, promiscuous sexual behaviour with a long line of partners can also be an indication (as it can in adults) that things are going psychologically astray. It may be that they are on some long search for love and attention perceived as absent in their childhood; or, in the case of girls, it may be a re-enactment of some earlier abuse, and either the only way they've found 'love' in the past or a constant confirmation that they are without value. In her life-changing book, *Women Who Love Too Much*, Robin Norwood describes how young women especially may set off on a course of relationships with a series of inappropriate males (alcoholics, addicts, abusers, etc.) in order to make things right for them, as a way of controlling and compensating for the things they couldn't fix for their parents in their childhood.

Sexual matters are very value-laden – what seems the norm for one person is extreme for another – and it's not for me to say what's all right in sexual behaviour for young people and what's clearly a problem, but extremes of both disinterest or promiscuity (especially with unpleasant partners) may indicate that at least minimal help could save the young person from secret misery. Finally, while being homosexual has absolutely no connection with psychological disorders, having to hide it from one's family and friends can cause untold unhappiness. It's never easy for parents to learn that their son or daughter is gay, not least because they feel sad knowing the suffering that an intolerant society can cause, but in order to maintain a loving relationship that will last both of you into the future, it's important to be as accepting as you are able. If young people admit to being gay, you can be pretty sure they're right: it takes an awful lot of courage to 'come out' and it's very unlikely that they've made a mistake or that they can change.

THE PSYCHOLOGICAL EFFECTS OF PHYSICAL DISEASE

Having even a short-term illness will often disturb children briefly, but with chronic illness such as diabetes, muscular dystrophy, kidney failure or deafness children and adolescents may go through various difficult stages as they become aware of and learn to cope with their disability. There may often be periods of depression or, more usually, of 'bad' behaviour. It is quite common for adolescents with diabetes to get out of control with their insulin, and psychological help as well as medical, will be most useful as a way of letting the young person come to terms with the problems. Similarly, a recent article by Sluckin* described the case of James, a young boy who, in addition to fairly abominable behaviour, was putting at risk his newly transplanted kidney. His psychologist helped him, via his drawings (see Figure 6) and writing, to say goodbye properly to his old kidney, and to accept the new one. He also helped the parents to provide some of the attention that James had lost now he no longer needed to use a kidney machine; and explored with the boy his anxieties about mixing with other children, anxieties that made him behave badly towards them before they did to him.

HYPERACTIVITY

Apart from a very high level of over-activity (dashing around, touching, grasping, investigating objects with unusual speed and intensity and often destructive power), children who are hyperactive are also very impulsive and easily distracted, with very short attention spans. They seem to lack fear and be very excitable, and may have slight coordination problems and some learning difficulties. They pester, and nag for their own way, and often seem

* Sluckin, A. (1986). Gestalt therapy and renal failure. *Changes*, *4*, 232.

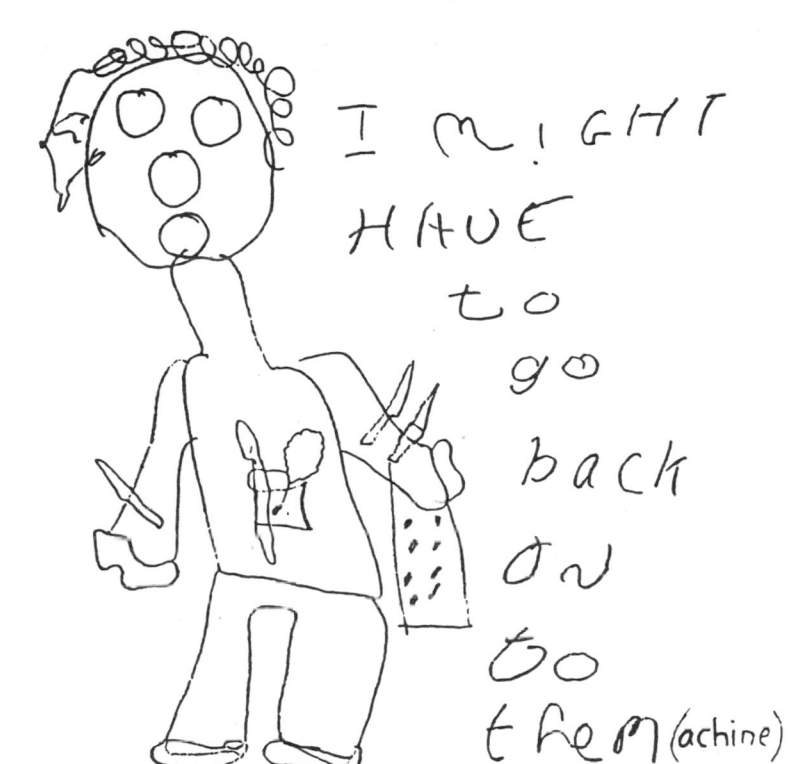

Fig. 6: 'I might have to go back on to the machine'

clearly out of control. Sometimes the child isn't actually more active, but the disorganised way he or she approaches tasks makes it appear so.

In Britain this condition is diagnosed very rarely: the proportion is generally said to be around three per cent, compared to the US where up to 20 per cent of pre-school children are said to be suffering from the problem. The enormous differences are probably due to variation in what it takes to make a diagnosis, rather than any cultural differences between the two countries. The main symptom, hyperactivity, is very disruptive of both home and school, and parents and teachers will consider they have a hyperactive child on their hands far more often than it will be actually diagnosed. This will often occur where a bright toddler is getting too little attention for its needs. Certainly if hyperactivity occurs only in the home or in the school, rather than in both, the diagnosis would not be applied in Britain. At the same time, if the parents are at their wits' end because of the child's terribly difficult behaviour, the fact that it only happens at home doesn't make it any less of a problem for them: in such cases whether a diagnosis would be given or not hardly seems important!

There has been a long debate about whether this syndrome (a group of behaviours, rather than an illness) is the result of some brain damage, or not. A recent review of the disorder came to the conclusion, however, that there was no firm evidence for even minimal damage. There is, however, some possibility that the disorder may be linked to difficult births, but it's quite likely that such a baby will behave differently from others after its trauma, and it may be that this behaviour has an effect on the way the parents react to their unexpectedly difficult baby, which may in turn encourage some of the less attractive features of its behaviour, and so on.

Children are sometimes given drug treatment for hyperactivity: either small doses of the major tranquilliser chlorpromazine, or more usually some form of stimulant such as Ritalin (or 'speed'). That stimulants are more successful than placebos in children who already appear over-stimulated seems very strange. But the theory of their success lies in the possibility that these children are actually *under*-stimulated (either environmentally or physiologically, in some way) and that raising their internal level of stimulation stops them having to dash around 'seeking a high' – or possibly that 'speed' simply increases their concentration. However, drug treatment that goes on for years is never a happy solution for children, and a large proportion do not respond at all. Many workers feel therefore that psychological treatments which are often successful and carry none of the dangers or side-effects of drugs, should be the treatment of first choice or should be used alongside drug treatment. These behavioural therapies take several forms, such as rewarding children for longer and longer attention spans and focussing on single tasks, as well as exercises to help them keep more and more of their bodies still or able to move more slowly. Changing children's diets was regarded as a possible method of cure, but the evidence to support its success has been disappointing.

Most of the evidence to date suggests that hyperactivity fades by adolescence, though some of the concentration and behaviour problems may remain and social, psychological and educational effects may be longer lasting.

TICS

These are sudden involuntary movements of muscles. They most commonly affect the face, and especially cause eye-blinking, but may also cause exaggerated movements of the head and neck, or include the whole top half of the body. Occasionally children have vocal tics – sudden unintentional noises or words.

In one survey about five per cent of seven-year-olds, mainly boys, had had tics at some stage or another, but there are fewer as children get older. No one knows how they are caused, although they're often thought to be 'nervous' in origin. Certainly children who suffer from tics show more of the anxiety problems of childhood described above; however, it must be very tough for a child to have to suffer from a problem so difficult to hide from his peers, and it's not surprising if these children are found to be showing rather more signs of distress. Whatever the cause, tics usually improve with age, and almost half have vanished completely within a few years.

SCHIZOPHRENIA

This condition is described in detail in Chapter 13. While its diagnosis is quite common in late adolescence, it is extremely rare for any of its more classic aspects to appear before adolescence at the earliest, and any diagnosis made before that time would be very unusual. Before puberty children can sometimes react to stress in dramatic ways which resemble schizophrenia, distinguishing fantasy and reality with difficulty, having terrifying nightmares and sometimes problems knowing who they are. They may become preoccupied with death and disaster, and this may show in their drawings and stories.

Although such often bizarre behaviour is very upsetting to parents, if there has been clear emotional stress in the child's life (for example, moving to a new town or school, losing or fearing to lose someone close, family upheavals, and so on) then chances are the problem will be short-lived with help going either directly to the child, in terms of psychotherapy, or by family therapy. Very occasionally drug treatment will be given.

It should also be remembered that children often hallucinate (see things that aren't there) when they have a fever, or occasionally after a general anaesthetic at the dentist's where frightening dreams may continue into reality for a few hours. Occasionally people report that earlier experimentation with drugs such as LSD, glue, or magic mushrooms, which are hallucinogenic (cause you to see or hear things which aren't present in reality), have had a disturbing effect for years afterwards, especially if the hallucinations produced were very frightening. These effects usually reappear only when the person is very tired or troubled by various stresses and may only last for an evening and gradually become more and more infrequent over months or years.

If an adolescent has a full psychotic breakdown, as described in Chapter 13, a similar pattern of behaviours to those discussed above may occur and, at this age, it is more likely to be diagnosed and treated as adult schizophrenia. Nevertheless, really 'mad' breakdowns can happen to anyone under extreme stress and so, if this has been evident, the stress itself should be dealt with wherever possible. In addition, recent research shows that family therapy which aims at encouraging parents to be less protective and less critical, is also a very useful way of preventing young people from having a second breakdown. Whether or not drug treatment will continue alongside other forms of therapy should depend on how well the young person is seen to manage without it.

THE CAUSES OF PSYCHOLOGICAL PROBLEMS IN CHILDREN

One of the most enduring debates in psychology is how much of our character and intelligence we inherit from our parents, and how much we acquire from growing up with them. This is the nature/nurture debate and, although there are no neat answers, it's clear that both factors are going to have a strong effect on how we are throughout our lives. Most of the research uses twin studies where identical twins grow up together or where they have been adopted into different homes: this allows likenesses and differences in behaviour to be compared in both groups. Generally results suggest that twins reared separately are not so alike as those reared together, but more alike than other siblings brought up apart, indicating that both nature and nurture has an effect: both the baby's temperament and its environment are important.

But even identical twins reared apart from birth have still shared the same environment for the nine months their mother was pregnant, and this intra-uterine period has been shown to have effects on later health and behaviour. For example, it's common knowledge now that smoking during pregnancy has an adverse effect upon the babies: they're often smaller and they cry more frequently. In a survey which followed 16,000 children from birth to adulthood, the children of mothers who smoked heavily during pregnancy were less well adjusted socially at the age of seven.

This shows the problems of trying to decide whether something is inherited or acquired. But there are even more subtle ways that the two aspects become blended. Children probably inherit some aspects of personality from their parents – some are more anxious than others, some seem to get depressed more easily – but, once again, it's difficult to decide whether this is actually inherited or whether it comes from growing up with anxious or depressed parents whose characteristics they share. Moreover, it's difficult to say what we mean by 'anxious' or 'depressed' in young children, let alone in babies. Generally, we're looking for behavioural clues like how much they cry, how much they sleep, or smile, or play, how much they eat, and so on.

Research has shown that on these small behavioural signs babies differ enormously, and probably largely genetically (though again a baby who's had a rough time in the womb or during birth is probably going to cry more and sleep less on a whole than one who hasn't). On their own none of these signs would lead to psychological problems, of course; where things can go wrong is that most of us as parents react differently to the different baby behaviours. Of course, we'd rather have a child who smiles a lot than one who doesn't; it makes us feel we're doing a good job. Of course, it's much easier and also more gratifying to have a good sleeper and one that doesn't cry too much, both because it means we get less tired and so we're happier when we do interact with the baby, and also again because we feel that this is what should happen. If it doesn't happen, the doubts creep in that maybe we're doing something wrong. The mother reacts more anxiously or more grumpily to the baby who undoubtedly notices it and cries more, and so the cycle may continue, perhaps getting worse throughout the pre-school years and even beyond.

Babies even differ in how well they can suck, and such an apparently tiny variation can have an enormous effect on the mother-child relationship, especially if the mother is breastfeeding. If the baby sucks well (but not so well that it hurts) the mother will feel she's doing a wonderful job, producing good nourishing milk, and so on. She will feel very warm to her baby in response, and the baby will feel safe and relaxed with her. If it sucks poorly she is quite likely to blame herself initially, and then feel angry; mealtimes will become anxious right from the beginning. If the mother feels inadequate rather than accepting that her baby is slightly different from the norm, the relationship between them may never be quite as easy and relaxed as between the good sucker and its mum. And of course, both children may be in the same family, so comparisons are made from day one!

This is not to be dismal or pessimistic about the future of some of our children; just the reverse. First, the important thing to remember and to be stressed both in the media and in the baby books, is that babies are *all* different – there's no absolutely correct group of behaviours. Second, it's the babies that are born with these differences; on their own they don't matter, and they're certainly not anybody's fault. If you can really believe this, then you are free to accept your baby and all its eccentricities, and love it for what it is rather than how well it conforms to the norms you've been led to believe. Of course, if you've got one that cries a lot, you'll be waking more in the night, but even this is not so bad if you don't secretly blame yourself for being wrong in some way.

How much any of this affects future relationships with the maturing child or adolescent is, of course, not known. The research involved would be impossibly difficult because every tiny interaction between them would need to be recorded to see how relationships really develop. However, I think it is very important in setting the groundwork for the relationship and for affecting the ways that both the child and the parents react to the different things that life throws up.

It's clear from most of this chapter that there are numerous aspects of a child's relationship with its parents that will have an effect on its psychological adjustment. There are the difficulties of having a depressed, anxious, obsessional parent, perhaps because the child will feel responsible for making things OK. There is the problem of having one who is absent, especially through sickness or divorce or death, because of the guilt and anger this can raise in the child. There are difficulties that can be caused for the child by a sibling who is chronically ill or dies. Then there's the whole arena of family allegiances: the son who is used as support by the mother against the father; the father who has incest with his daughter so making impossible a bond between her and her mother; the child who carries all the problems of the family as a scapegoat.

Families are places where good things happen and also bad things. This is the case in every family. The problems don't come about because bad things happen so much as because we pretend that they don't. We make up all sorts of family myths and mottos which the child has to accept, even though they probably originate from our own families and may clearly not be true: 'In this family no one gets angry'; 'In this family we all love each other all the time'; 'In this family none of the children are ever jealous or envious'; 'Mummy and daddy are a perfect couple (despite the screaming matches you may think you overheard)'. And so on. What family therapy does, perhaps more than other forms, is to look at these myths and test them with the obvious reality, and let people try out ways of relating that don't involve pretence.

I am very aware of talking of parents as the cause of many of their children's problems. What one must also bear in mind is that parents and children live in a society and an environment which causes innumerable stress and problems for them both. One diagnostic system recognises general environmental stresses for children and categorises them as shown in Figure 7.

If your child is subjected to any of these or other stressors, it's perfectly normal for them to react in some way – in fact it will be abnormal if they don't. It might be physical, so they experience new aches and pains, or emotional so they begin to behave 'badly' or become very quiet, even mute, or clinging, etc. Alice, for

Stress level	Example
Minimal	Vacation with family
Mild	Change in school teacher; new school year
Moderate	Chronic parental fighting; change to new school; illness of close relative; birth of sibling
Severe	Death of peer; divorce of parents; arrest; admission to hospital; persistent, harsh parental discipline
Extreme	Death of parent or sibling; repeated physical or sexual abuse
Catastrophic	Multiple family deaths

Fig. 7: Examples of childhood stressors

example, when she was three, had been in hospital with pneumonia. After the first couple of days when she was obviously upset at being separated from her parents, she became very quiet and well behaved. When she was discharged after a week, she was quiet and cold for about a day, shrugging off her mum's cuddles, and for the next week was dreadfully badly behaved, smashing her little sister's toys and squashing the 'welcome home' cake her mum had baked. It took a lot of tolerance and lip-biting on her mother's part to continue to show her only love and affection, despite all this. Eventually Alice got into a rage over something and then suddenly burst into tears and let her mother comfort and cuddle her back to normal. It could have marked a change for the worse in their relationship but, thanks to her mother's understanding, it may well have brought them closer together.

School too can produce a lot of stress for children that's not always forgotten when they become adults. For example, while it's often recorded that children have made suicide attempts because of school bullies, I am also constantly amazed by the number of adult male clients I have had who still become engulfed with helpless fury at the memory of their gym teacher's humiliating behaviour towards them.

TREATMENT IN CHILDHOOD
AND ADOLESCENCE

One of the best aspects of working with children is that they respond so well to treatment: things *can* be changed relatively quickly for most of them, since they're still flexible. The difficulties arise from the rigidity of some parents, schools and social and housing environments which may all act to reduce the chance of change.

Individual psychotherapy is used by many therapists, perhaps involving play with dolls, or drawing, writing or acting out the problem. This may be most appropriate where the child has had some trauma, or where family relationships are difficult (for example, where a sibling is chronically ill, or there's been a divorce). It's also good for children who are physically ill in some way and having difficulty coming to terms with it. It's less useful in adolescence, where family therapy is often preferable.

Behaviour therapy is perhaps the most used treatment for children, and parents are commonly taught how to apply its methods; for example, giving rewards (attention, cuddles, a weekly treat) for behaviours which gradually come closer and closer to the goal.

Family therapy is used where relationships within the family need changing, and where all the family members agree. Although it takes some courage to 'behave' as a family in front of a stranger, when communication is stuck it's usually only someone who's uninvolved who can see objectively what's going wrong and provide some strategies for change. Although the changes won't be easy, it's rarely just the 'problem' child or adolescent who benefits in the end.

Drug treatment is generally not recommended for children. Although all the drugs that are used for adults may be used occasionally for children, they are all powerful and no one really knows what unwanted effects they have on someone who's still developing. One of the commonest prescribed is Tofranil, an antidepressant drug used for bedwetting. Since it may produce a number of problematic side-effects, and since its benefits for bedwetting only last while the drug is being taken and are, in any case, not as great as the buzzer, it's main use is to provide an easy temporary way to reduce embarrassment for the child if, for example, it is known that a visit or a holiday is to take place. In regard to more general use, a recent psychiatric review by Kaplan and Kolvin concluded that 'there is a lack of evidence of the efficacy of antidepressants in the prepubertal depressive disorders of childhood.'

The side-effects of the major tranquillisers make them generally unsuitable for children, especially as there is an extra risk of convulsions in the young. However, they will often be prescribed in adolescents when a diagnosis of schizophrenia has been given, and usually in this case at least brief hospitalisation will also be involved. Occasionally minor tranquillisers such as Valium are given to help a young person over an anxious event (for example, the return to school in a child who's been refusing to go), but they should only be taken for a very limited time and usually will go alongside one of the forms of therapy described above. Most people involved with helping children agree that psychological therapies are much more effective than drugs in the long run, with fewer risks. In addition, they are less likely to allow children (or their families) to view themselves as sick, and so to refuse responsibility for change.

Hospitalisation for emotional problems is rare in children but may be used briefly in cases of soiling, for example. In adolescents a period in a good centre may sometimes give them a chance to get away from family difficulties for long enough to begin to work through their anxieties and take the first necessary steps in separation. If possible it's useful if family therapy takes place at the same time.

Local self-help groups exist in some places for the young people themselves, including those for the children of alcoholics (Alateen) and for the victims of sexual abuse and for diabetes sufferers. In London and most large cities there are counselling services for young people such as the London Youth Advisory Centre (13 to 25) and the Tavistock Clinic for those who are older (16 to 30). The Brook Advisory Centres offer advice on sexual problems. There are also groups for parents of disturbed children (for example, autistic or hyperactive) which can be very supportive, and the NSPCC has groups to help parents who are feeling isolated. If as a parent you are suffering more than you feel is normal from your adolescent son or daughter, enquire to see if there's a parents' support group locally and, if there isn't, think seriously about starting one. Apart from often finding that things are no worse in your family than anyone else's, you can evolve strategies between you for dealing with the inevitable problems, and situations that seemed bleak when you were alone can seem almost funny when you swap your stories.

Chapter

12

The psychological problems of ageing

People in the later years of life enjoy the same pleasures and confront the same problems that younger people do. Most cope well, but a proportion will, of course, suffer from any of the problems of living described in other parts of this book. They may be anxious or obsessional; they perhaps have eating problems or become psychotic, often with paranoid fears; they may also become depressed. Although you can recognise the problems in much the same way as you can for those who are younger, some of the issues involved are a little different. Just as children's problems are sometimes dismissed by the idea that they're resilient, so too older people's difficulties are too often seen as due entirely to age, to being confused or to dementia.

Anxiety states are more common in the elderly than in any other age group. They are subject to the same rapid change in the world around them that we all are, but, because they're not taking such an active part in it, they can feel particularly helpless to the stress it causes: fears are so much worse if you feel you can do nothing about them. And there are real, more specific, fears too: that your money will run out, that you'll be robbed, that your constipation means cancer, that you may have to choose between warmth and food this winter, that your children will 'put you in a home', and so on. Moving into a pleasant old people's home is of course not necessarily a bad thing in itself, but the passivity and helplessness it implies is what hurts more: choosing to go into a home is one thing, but being put there is quite different.

Although many older people are 'content with their lot' and can face the fact that they will die with equanimity, a proportion become increasingly fearful of death and worry themselves, their relatives and their doctors constantly about their health. Chapter 7 discusses hypochondria and points out that reassurance is not the best approach to reduce the constant worrying: its effects are short-lived and the anxiety returns as much as or more than before. It's often much more useful to talk about the actual fear or depression that's underlying the concern with their bodies and what this means to the person, rather than dismissing it or insisting on yet another distressing investigation. Similarly, obsessional behaviour may also develop in the elderly as a means of reducing anxiety: a fear of being robbed or murdered in their beds can prompt endless checking and re-checking of locks and windows and can mean that sleep is reduced still further.

Many people become more paranoic as they grow older (see p. 206). Of course, trusting people less can be quite a protection nowadays, and is positively encouraged in the elderly with advertisements urging them not to let people into their homes without first checking their identity. This is completely necessary but it's only another step on for people to decide they can't trust the identity cards themselves and so not let anyone in at all, not even the health visitor or the social worker. One more step and the doctor, called by the worries of the health visitor, is also refused entry. He can see through the letter-box the need for physical and psychological help and calls the psychiatrist who has to get the social workers and police to help force an entry so compulsory hospital care can be provided.

This is of course fictitious, but it lets you see how even psychotic states of paranoic delusions – where the old person is convinced that 'they' are out to get him or her – may have their roots very firmly in the realities of their environment and in society as a whole. Albert, in his late eighties, was living with his daughter and, over the past few months had begun to accuse her of poisoning his food. She cared for him and loved him a lot and felt enormously upset by these accusations.

I was convinced Dad was beginning to dement. He seemed to be acting so peculiarly to me, and he was so jealous of Tony, my boyfriend. The trouble was that every time anyone came to see him, he was as nice as pie: there seemed to be no problem at all. My doctor put me on to a social worker who came and talked to us both separately, and later on together. He asked me on my own whether it wasn't true that I would be much better off when my father had gone; he realised that I was postponing getting married because of Dad. He let me see it was quite OK to admit this – it didn't mean I loved Dad any the less.

When they all talked together her father was at last able to bring up his guilt about still being alive and, when the fear that she would 'get rid of him' (or put him in a home) was really aired, the paranoic symptoms disappeared. It's so much better to address the fears when they arise, rather than treating them as nonsense so that the person feels left more and more alone with their terror.

Another commonsense (but often overlooked) reason for growing feelings of paranoia in the elderly is the deafness that increases with age and that makes life more frightening, especially as people are not always aware they're growing deaf. A hearing aid works wonders!

Most people do have the resources and the strength, both physical and psychological, to feel very good about themselves as they grow older, and in fact self-esteem has been shown to increase with age. Nevertheless, depression in the elderly is still very common. It may show the same picture of sadness and crying and apathy, or the deadness where movement and motivation is completely absent so that they cease caring even for their most basic needs. It may also appear in a very agitated form with tremendous anxiety and pacing up and down and wringing of hands. All the causes discussed in Chapter 6 apply but some, such as learned helplessness, loss and social causes are more obvious in the later years.

Although many people can live to a ripe old age and suffer no more losses than anyone else, the chances of close relatives and friends dying is of course much greater. Quite often we are more able to be philosophical about bereavement as we grow older, but sometimes people do get stuck at one of the stages of grieving (pp. 32–5). Other losses, often given less thought than actual death, are of property, youth, pets, income, security, good health and energy, work and status.

All the treatments discussed for the psychological problems described in the rest of the book are also used in older people. In the more serious forms of depression, for example, you will often need to go into hospital and the treatment may be largely anti-depressants and ECT. Both can sometimes lift your mood when depression is severe but, if it keeps returning, it's better not to have repeated courses of ECT. Physical treatments like these are used proportionally more than psychotherapy in older people. This is perhaps because of a myth (actually emphasised by Freud!) that older people find it more difficult to change. More recent research has shown that you can quite successfully 'teach an old dog new tricks' of living, and various forms of psychotherapy – exploratory, behavioural and cognitive – have all proved to be helpful.

The issues that are specifically concerned with ageing and which often emerge in exploratory psychotherapy are feelings of dissatisfaction with what they have achieved, or that life suddenly seems a bit like a pointless exercise. In those who have recently retired or been made redundant, they may feel they don't know how to act now that their 'false self' – the one they've used at work and at home over so many years – is no longer needed. Therapy then becomes a search for the lost self – the one they left behind when they were children. They often see difficulty in new aspects of their close relationships; for example, that their children have begun to mother them, rather than vice-versa.

Many men find that, as they grow older, they become less aggressively masculine and admit to new needs for dependence and tenderness, traditionally seen as feminine. Most men enjoy the wider experiences this allows, but others find the needs frightening and upsetting. Women too tend to change in the opposite direction, often finding themselves able to act more aggressively and independently, and some of them may again find this is a bit scary, especially if their husbands are now appearing in more need of security and seeming more dependent. This does not represent any physical change – we all have both sets of characteristics within us. It's more that, within set roles laid down by society, our repressed side begins to emerge.

Valerie was 57 and her doctor wrote that she had seemed depressed and anxious ever since suffering from salmonella poisoning. She was a very 'proper' person, full of rules about how life should be lived, and how close one human being (her) should let herself be to another (me). She seemed to see the salmonella as a failure – socially and physically – and felt dirty and anxious as a result. Despite her continuing ill-health, she was doing extremely well in the company in which she'd worked ever since she'd left her husband eight years earlier, unable any longer to tolerate his drunkenness. However, now she declared she couldn't be bothered to go on getting any higher. She blamed her depression on the grief she couldn't seem to shake off since her little dog had died.

Over the course of therapy we began to discuss her anxiety over the feelings of independence and self-sufficiency she was starting to experience now her last child was leaving home. She had every right to start enjoying herself, but somehow she couldn't quite allow it to happen. We talked a lot about loss, starting with her dog and leading to her husband (for all his faults), her parents, and her children who'd now all left home. Letting herself grieve for these seemed to free her in a way that allowed her to begin competing once more at work, and her depression clearly lifted.

We looked too at her concern with 'dirtiness' and 'bad behaviour' and after some time she confessed, with shame, that she had had a 'one night stand' shortly before the salmonella. She seemed to feel she was being punished for experiencing any sort of sexual needs or pleasure. Much of the therapy was concerned with getting her to give herself permission both to have sexual needs for as long as she wanted, and to explore them within the relationship she eventually began with a colleague. Her anxiety symptoms left her gradually over the course of therapy.

Behaviour therapies can also be used very successfully with older clients; for example, by using diaries and other means to work out ways of increasing pleasant events and decreasing unpleasant ones. What gives you pleasure is not presumed (and surprisingly not always really known by you!) but is discovered by tracking which activities improve or lower your mood over a few weeks. Lily, whom we talked about on page 87, was helped in this way once she'd begun to get herself dressed and to respond to people once more. Keeping a diary in hospital encouraged her to attend events there she might otherwise have missed – just so she had something to write about! She learnt that she really enjoyed the yoga class, discovered old skills in ballroom dancing, loved having her hair done at the hairdressers and had an unexpected talent for table tennis. When she was discharged, many of these activities were located for her by the social worker in her neighbourhood and, a year later, she was still content and enjoying quite an active social life.

Being taught and practising relaxation has been found to reduce anxiety levels in elderly people, and assertiveness training lets them feel less helpless and reduces depression. Cognitive therapy, which teaches you to challenge old rules and beliefs which are inappropriate and may be causing you unnecessary unhappiness, is also used widely, and this has been shown to reduce both anxiety and depression in elderly people as well as the young.

Group therapy is also common, particularly in hospitals, and breaks down some of the barriers and difficulties older people may find in relating to one another; while helping each other lets them feel useful once again – a feeling that's too often denied people both in hospital and in the community.

THE DEMENTIAS

True dementias are organic diseases – that is, they are the result of actual physical changes in the brain – and it's beyond the scope of this book to deal with them in any detail. There are a number of causes, some of which are treatable, and so great care is needed to see which type of dementia is being suffered. Those that can possibly be treated include some which are caused by alcohol or drugs or poisons, others which are due to conditions such as hypoglycaemia or vitamin B12 deficiency or various tumours. However, for the two which are most common – Alzheimer's disease and multi-infarct dementia – there is still no cure.

Multi-infarct dementia causes between 10 and 20 per cent of cases and comes from a series of small strokes which injure small areas of the brain. There is not the gradual loss of functioning that occurs in Alzheimer's, but things get worse in steps, often staying the same for quite a while in between. Both dementias show the same signs of increasing memory loss and intellectual deterioration.

We have no idea of the cause of Alzheimer's disease but it's responsible for around 60 per cent of dementias – which amounts to around half a million people in Britain alone. Although it generally starts in people older than 65 (senile dementia), it can begin as young as 45 (pre-senile dementia). It usually has a slow beginning with signs which may initially resemble psychological problems: sleeping may become erratic, they may be agitated and anxious or seem depressed. Sometimes they show strong signs of paranoia or jealousy. However, it's worth remembering Albert's situation above, and also that delirium rather than dementia can cause confusion and sometimes many quite wild symptoms, including paranoia and hallucinations (see p. 98). The next stage shows clear memory problems and other intellectual difficulties, and this is often followed by a period of 'withdrawal', a deadening of spontaneous behaviour. They may have more specific problems such as difficulty in finding the right word for something, or understanding people, or repeating things over and over, or remembering what an object like a refrigerator is used for. The course of the illness runs between five and ten years with gradual physical deterioration including incontinence.

Certain conditions can produce behaviours very much like dementia. For example, severe constipation can make older people clearly confused. Similarly, depression in the elderly is very often mistaken for dementia. Because Alzheimer's is still not curable, but depression is, it's extremely important to make sure which condition the person is actually suffering from. If they're relatively young there's a tendency to see the symptoms as depression, but if they're over 60 dementia might be the thing that springs to mind. Deciding which it is is generally done by elaborate testing, especially of memory, usually by a neuro-psychologist, or by a psychiatrist or neurologist. However, there are a few signs that give you a clue: as a relative, you can usually be fairly precise about when the depression began, whereas the start of Alzheimer's is more difficult to pinpoint; people with depression usually complain about their memory and concentration problems, both short-term and long-term, whereas those with Alzheimer's are often oblivious that they have any problems, and memory is usually worse for recent events; depressed people are more likely to say 'don't know' in reply to questions about events, whereas those with Alzheimer's will make near-miss answers; while those with depression will quickly lose their social skills, people with Alzheimer's may hang on to the niceties of social interaction for quite some time, though there may also be the occasional large blunder.

Although there is no curative treatment for Alzheimer's disease or for multi-infarct dementia, there are many forms of psychological therapies which will make the course of the illness more tolerable for the sufferers, particularly by working with their relatives who are inevitably placed under enormous strain, sometimes for a number of years.

Help for families

The most useful first step if you have a close relative diagnosed as suffering from dementia is to gather together all the information you can about the particular problem; for example, by reading books and pamphlets on the subject or by finding out from organisations such as Age Concern or MIND or the Alzheimer's Disease Society. Voluntary bodies like the Samaritans will usually have the addresses of local groups and services which may provide information, support and relief for holidays or days off.

Many of the problems for relatives are made worse by the fact that the roles they're used to (for example, mother and daughter) have changed full-face and that someone they'd looked to perhaps for advice and support now acts like a small child. For example, they may repeat the same question over and over. It is better to have the knowledge that this, and the resulting anxiety and confusion, is only a result of memory loss; it's not done to spite, or because she or he never listens to you, and there's really nothing you can do by way of exercises that will substantially improve the person's memory. If a person is having trouble finding the word for an object, however, it is often possible to get them to describe it with a number of words; forcing them to try to remember will only make them more anxious, and anxiety will make their problems worse.

These problems of changing roles include those where we judge an activity (such as looking at a child's picture book or watching TV all day) as beneath the dignity of the parent or spouse we used to know. Accepting that the person's happiness is the main thing and that past evaluations of worthwhile pursuits are simply no longer relevant will often let you react with affection rather than irritation at these behaviours.

Behaviour therapy can often help you to work out better daily schedules for elderly persons. For example, a common complaint is that they are up half the night wandering around; however, a careful analysis of their day's activities often reveals that they spend a lot of it cat-napping or even sleeping quite soundly: it's not surprising they find it hard to sleep at night! And now you can do something about it.

Looking after a demented relative is undoubtedly stressful, and so you should take every care to look after yourself too and to take part in any stress-reducing activities you can (see Chapter 3), and keep up at least one outside hobby or sport or entertainment. It's quite likely that you'll feel even more burdened if you think that it's only you, rather than other members of your family, who are left responsible for your relative. Actually meeting with the other family members and working out acceptable ways for them to share the load – even if it's only occasionally – will help to relieve your anger and so make the caretaking seem less distressing. Books on assertion training such as *Your Perfect Right*, and *Don't Say 'Yes' When You Want To Say 'No'*, may give you good strategies to get round particularly difficult family members.

Support groups of others in your position are enormously helpful, both to enable you to share a good moan and perhaps too a good laugh, and also to provide information and advice from similar experiences, as well as cover for each other. If there isn't one handy, you should think seriously about starting one yourself. Bring in outside help whenever it is available or as often as you can afford it. Women often find it particularly difficult to bring in someone to look after their husbands, feeling guilty that they're unable to provide the nonstop help he needs; men, on the other hand, rarely see this as a problem. A mixed support group can therefore share experiences which will relieve feelings such as guilt. Cilla joined an informal local group whose members were the caretakers of relatives suffering any form of dementia.

I felt quite nervous of saying what was going on for me at first. I was a real turmoil of emotions. I think the thing I get most from them now I've grown to know them and seen their own problems, is that I can show my feelings as openly as I want: not bottling things up has made me feel better in myself, even physically fitter. I had a good cry in front of them when I could finally admit how sad I was to 'lose' the man I'd married. Once I'd done that I found it so much easier to care for Tom as he is now. And sometimes I have a real roar about the unfairness of it all. We get in guest speakers too occasionally, and one night we had a workshop on assertion training – how to get what you need from the council or from relatives! Above all we find that together we can have a laugh, and that's probably the most valuable thing of all.

Chapter

Psychosis and the schizophrenias

Richard arrived at the door with an old friend of mine who asked if he could come in to play my piano; he'd just arrived back from the Middle East and hadn't played for so long. My piano was slightly out of tune, but that didn't account for the extraordinary harmonies and disharmonies that came out of the music room. I couldn't decide if he was a genius or if he was playing the fool; or was it both? I'd just made a cake and offered him some; apart from our own small slices he ate the rest. He explained that he'd not been eating at home because his parents were poisoning him by feeding him flour made from the bones of ground-up Iranians. In a monologue that darted from topic to topic he mentioned he'd shot the Shah. I told him I'd seen the Shah on TV just that day. A cardboard cut-out, he retorted. He added that the Iranian and British police had agreed to use this model in order to lure him into a false sense of security. He stopped talking occasionally in mid-sentence to listen (I later realised) to the voices which told him what was happening. As he spoke he looked down at my son's first music book:

'GBDF,' Richard read the title out loud. 'Ground Bones Deliver Food, that's what it stands for,' he concluded instantly. 'Then again', he added, with a laugh at the wall, rather than at our nonplussed faces, 'It might just stand for the musical notes that pass through the lines.'

Richard was taken to hospital later that day by his parents and their GP. He stayed there three months and, when I visited him, he admitted that he could still hear the voices talking to him but he now told the doctors they were silent. He realised he'd be discharged more readily when the voices had gone away.

He was right to think that auditory hallucinations were seen as a vital symptom. In a famous study back in 1973 by Rosenhan in the States, a group of researchers presented themselves individually at 12 psychiatric hospitals and complained simply of hearing voices which said 'empty' and 'hollow' and 'thud', not always very clearly. All but one of them were promptly given the diagnosis of schizophrenia and admitted to hospital for an average of almost three weeks. They were discharged with the diagnosis of 'schizophrenia in remission'.

This study's findings were, of course, very embarrassing to anyone holding firm ideas about psychiatric diagnosis, and I'll discuss the implications for this shortly. But they also illustrate the point that 'hearing voices' is regarded as a prime symptom indicating schizophrenia. In fact, far more common amongst people who are suffering from a schizophrenia-type disorder is a state of disorganised thinking such as Richard showed, where you're unable to get your thoughts together in any coherent way. One thought flashes to another in a bizarre way that switches between sense and nonsense to anyone listening: the wisdom and the wit and the pathos of Shakespeare's fools offer some idea of this.

Basically, you're likely to be given a diagnosis of schizophrenia if, firstly, you act strangely, either very chaotically or particularly bizarrely, or, alternatively, if you don't show any spontaneous behaviour at all. The latter condition is called 'catatonic' schizophrenia, and nowadays is seen extremely rarely, but there is often a deadened look in someone with the more common disorder, with fear or laughter or surprise coming at times that seem inappropriate. Secondly, the diagnosis may be given if you seem very confused, with extremely disorganised ideas and especially with auditory hallucinations (voices) like Richard, or perhaps with delusions that you're someone you're not, where it becomes increasingly difficult to distinguish reality from fantasy and self from others. Having paranoic delusions that They are out to get you may be present or not. It's sometimes a consequence of the other symptoms; for example, the police may well be looking for

Richard if, as the voices had told him, he'd killed the Shah. You may feel that you're being controlled in some way by others, as Edward, described below, illustrates. All this can be, and usually is, very frightening and distressing, and occasionally may make you potentially dangerous either to yourself or to others.

Edward described what had happened to him very calmly. He told us how he had been sitting at the desk in the council office when he saw a group of Rebels and a group of Feds, the two sides of the American Civil War, rush towards each other and begin to battle. The detail of the fighting was intricate. Edward's fear and shouting and warnings as he'd ducked below desks and thrown objects at the soldiers had resulted in his being hospitalised and diagnosed as suffering from schizophrenia. Asked whether he believed he'd actually seen this take place in and among the desks while secretaries continued with their work, he answered:

'Of course I don't believe it was really happening. It's just more proof that they've put a transistor up at the back of my throat which they can operate whenever they like. They can make me think or see or hear anything they want to.'

He told us how he'd had his tonsils out when he was eight, and the transistor had obviously been planted then. The psychiatrist asked him if he really believed that the transistor was there: 'Of course. I have to believe it, don't I? If it's not true then it means I'm mad.'

Beliefs such as these are sufficiently abnormal to clearly indicate madness to most people. Although visual hallucinations (seeing things not there) are rare, taken with the notion of thought control, they may be enough to make a psychiatrist decide upon a diagnosis of schizophrenia.

It should be clear from all this that the one thing you certainly don't have is a 'split personality', despite the fact that many references to schizophrenia that are made in the media *still* seem to presume that this is the definition. The chaos that people so often experience with these disorders makes it clear that they are having great problems hanging on to even one coherent personality, let alone two or more. As I've said, violence is also seen occasionally if the hallucinations and delusions encourage enough fear.

Generally speaking, first schizophrenic breakdowns come when people are young, generally between the ages of 17 and 30, though diagnoses are made both younger and older than this. They occur more frequently in men than in women. For some people this will be a single event, lasting perhaps only a few weeks, while for others it will continue in some form throughout their lives.

In this chronic form, apathy and a lack of feelings (not always easy to distinguish from drug effects) can be extremely disabling, with some people finding no way again to hold a job or make lasting relationships. These are the men and women who formed most of the population of psychiatric hospitals, though who are increasingly being cared for within the community (of course, in some countries where 'craziness' is more easily tolerated, they have always stayed in the community) where, with proper help, they are often found to have more skills and need fewer drugs than before. With so much uncertainty involved in schizophrenia, it is never justified, even with the most crazy people, to see the disorder as irreversible or hopeless.

The acute form of schizophrenic breakdown is often in response to some stress or pressure. The description of Janet in Chapter 4, shows the way that very anxious feelings can build up uncontrollably until you need to alter the ways you see or experience things in order to explain what's happening or to find a way out. With the exhaustion that comes from not daring to sleep, we may crack up and let the awful perceptions and thoughts flood us so we can no longer recognise reality. Terrifying as this is, it's usually short-lived: in a review of studies of people hospitalised with a diagnosis of schizophrenia, O'Brien pointed out: 'Most individuals, under current conditions of treatment, may be expected to recover from their acute psychotic 'nervous breakdown' within four to eight weeks.'

As I said in the first chapter of this book, these disorders are called 'psychotic' (as opposed to neurotic) which implies that the behaviours that characterise them are different in quality from normal behaviour. The two principal conditions falling into the category of psychosis are the schizophrenias and manic-depression, although certain other depressions (for example, post-natal), reactions to severe stress in adolescents, and drug and alcohol disorders may also appear psychotic.

Certainly, most of us would see both of the men described above as abnormal in important aspects of their thoughts and behaviour: they were clearly not acting as most of us do, and their behaviour was making it difficult for them to operate in the everyday world.

At the same time, we all need to be constantly aware that what's regarded as normal or abnormal changes both over time and between different cultures within each society. So having grown up with a psychic relative, I've personally never doubted that people can be seen and talked to after they are dead. For this reason, I don't start instantly wondering if an old lady may be mad if all she describes is feeling and hearing her recently dead husband in the room with her. In fact this is a common reaction to grief but while some people would clearly see it as abnormal, for me it fits within my ideas of normality.

Of course, with abnormal thoughts and behaviours as a main criteria for diagnosis, things become particularly difficult when very different cultures are concerned; for example, various black cultures, or Moslem, or Japanese, can all show behaviours that seem quite abnormal to the usually white middle-class professionals who will be consulted on the subject, or who will write the text-books that will teach the next generation of professionals. The differences between cultures don't need to be even this wide, however, to bring about differences in what's normal and what isn't: it may happen between sexes and between classes. I recently read the following cases in a chapter on schizophrenia by Forrest, an eminent psychiatrist, which he used to illustrate the point that 'an alteration in functioning in the work situation, at school, at work . . .' could indicate schizophrenia.

Andy, aged 16 years, was due to sit his 'O' levels. He had one brother with a PhD and another with a promised place at University. Andy had entered for five subjects but only in fact sat the papers for three and passed two. He stopped going to school and started to become hostile and verbally aggressive towards his mother.

Sydney, aged 19 years, began to stay in bed all day and get up in the evening. He would cook himself a meal apart from the rest of the family late in the evening and then stay up half the night listening to his transistor.

Eddie is alleged to have been a quiet, normal boy before going to England for his National Service. When he was demobbed he got himself a labouring job but some months later he gave it up, stating that the means of production should be in the hands of the workers. After two

*months lying around the house his father threw him out and he went to
live in a lodging house.*

The author concludes these three 'presentations are fairly
characteristic of schizophrenia . . .' Obviously to people whose
children went to public school and so were spared such frustrations, these behaviours are abnormal, whereas to many of us
they are either normal illustrations of adolescence, or at worst,
show clear signs of unhappiness. Leaving a job because of the
Marxist statement that 'the means of production should be in the
hands of the workers' is unusual in this country, but on its own
only indicates strongly held political views. We know that
holding political views different from the majority is unacceptable in the Soviet Union, certainly before Gorbachov, and psychiatry is involved in trying to change these views. While this is
clearly an abuse of human rights, we obviously cannot be too
smug that we don't innocently do the same here. A few years
back the clear media vilification of Tony Benn as 'loony' (how
could a peer of the realm give up so much to bring about social
change for the benefit of the poor and not be mad?) shows the
way that unacceptable behaviour can be seen as abnormal to
some, and it's not unknown for a Rastafarian to be diagnosed as
schizophrenic because he believes Haile Selassie (as opposed to
Jesus) was the son of God.

Having sounded these warning bells, I accept that it may well
have been the case that these three boys did suffer from a
schizophrenia-type disorder; they may also have shown signs of
thought disorder or mind control or any of the other behaviours
described above. These disorders do not always appear dramatically, but sometimes there are changes in mood and behaviour
and performance which take place over months. I've used the
quotes merely to illustrate that there will always be cultural
differences between ideas of normality and abnormality which
may affect diagnosis.

I talked about the problem of diagnosis in the first chapter: the
ways that it can imply false certainty and narrow our vision in
regard to treatment and hope; also the way that the implication of
a specific 'mental illness' itself implies that this is something
lodged within the individual, rather than society or his or her
interaction with society. The labelling of someone as schizophre-

nic has more serious implications than most other diagnoses, and so the problems need considering in some detail.

There are some individuals whom most psychiatrists in the world would agree should be given the diagnosis of schizophrenia: they show enough of the key signs (for example, of thought disorder, hallucinations, inappropriate moods or thought control) while clearly not suffering from manic-depression (Chapter 14) or severe or agitated depression (Chapter 6) or any disease of the brain (such as a tumour or head injury) or a paranoid disorder (p. 206) or any condition related to drugs or alcohol. Whereas some doctors will see this as indicating that a clear illness called schizophrenia exists, others will take a less certain line and describe it as a residual category of psychosis – the rather rag-bag group of behaviours that are left after all these others have been ruled out. This is the line taken by the US psychiatrist, Patrick O'Brien, in his clear and useful book, *The Disordered Mind: What We Know About Schizophrenia*. Despite the title, he usually refers to the condition as 'schizophrenia-type disorders', and feels a really vague name such as 'unspecified psychosis' or 'psychosis of unknown origin' would be more useful.

Despite there being a sizeable proportion of individuals whom psychiatrists would clearly agree should be given this diagnosis, there is a similarly large proportion about whom there would be disagreement. Although the figure is commonly given that one person in every hundred suffers from schizophrenia and that these rates are fairly uniform around the world, there is also the fact that US doctors, for example, are far more likely to use the diagnosis than British doctors who, in a comparative study, were found to be more likely to call the same individuals manic-depressive.

Other studies have found that there was a sharp increase in the numbers diagnosed as schizophrenic when the major tranquillisers were introduced (there was at last something that could be done for schizophrenia), and a decrease when Lithium was introduced for manic-depression (again, there was now something that could be done for sufferers with that disorder). Because the difficulties of being sure of a diagnosis are well known, and because schizophrenia is a serious diagnosis to give to a person, initial psychotic breakdowns will rarely be labelled schizophrenic. This is especially important because breakdowns which last only a short time and have a sudden beginning have far less chance of relapse or of becoming chronic. They are given names such as acute psychotic or schizophrenic-type episode, as opposed to the 'chronic' disorder in which several of the signs will have been obvious for at least six months.

I can understand it if all this feels very frustrating. As I've said a number of times throughout this book, we all long for certainty in life – that's all of us including the doctors as well as those they treat. Life is insecure and chaotic enough for most of us, and we want to be able to trust and believe that the professionals at least have some of the answers. A clear-cut diagnosis provides relief for relatives and sometimes for the sufferers themselves. However, pretending that there is complete certainty when there is only some, is ultimately far more dangerous because it limits the ways we will think about the individual and his or her problems in the future: whether we think change is possible or whether drugs, for example, are always the best treatment, and so on.

THE CAUSES OF SCHIZOPHRENIC-TYPE DISORDERS

Like all of the disorders talked about in this book, the causes of this condition may be threefold: (1) People may have been born with the gene that inevitably or potentially will result in the problem, probably via a change in biochemistry. If this is so then we are more justified in calling it an illness; (2) They may suffer a physical change in their bodies, probably one which concerns their brain chemistry, and which results in the typical changes in mood and behaviour (again, if this were definitely the case, we would be describing an illness). (3) They may have life experiences, whether within the family or outside it, which affect them psychologically and perhaps physically to such an extent as to produce the disorder.

1) Genes and schizophrenia

There are usually one or two people in a family who can be pointed to as acting rather oddly, eccentrically, or at least differently to the rest of the family. If a young person in your family has been given a diagnosis of schizophrenia, it will be perfectly natural for you to look for such a black sheep, and often you'll be able to find one.

Medical science has also spent time and effort looking for a genetic basis to schizophrenia. If it exists, then it could act via the brain's chemistry, and so would lend weight to a biochemical model. The largest and most quoted study on the subject was conducted by Kallman using monozygotic and dizygotic (identical and non-identical) twins who had been adopted and one of whom had been diagnosed as suffering from schizophrenia. Kallman (whose early work on genetics had been conducted in Hitler's Germany) and his successors showed results which suggested that identical twins even reared separately were more likely to share the diagnosis than non-identical twins or other siblings.

These studies seemed to provide strong evidence that at least a predisposition to suffering from schizophrenia, if not the actual illness, was likely. This conclusion appears in most textbooks and is taught in most courses on psychiatry and psychology, despite the fact that over the past few years considerable doubt has been cast on the ways the findings were analysed, and even more fundamental problems have been raised (for example, by Rose, Kamin and Lewontin in *Not in our Genes*, and by Lidz and Blatt*). The French investigation by Cassou, Schiff and Stewart† in 1980 concluded: 'After a meticulous and exhaustive re-evaluation, we therefore conclude that there is no evidence for a genetic effect in the schizophrenic process.'

Once again I feel like apologising for the fact that there's still so much confusion and uncertainty. We grow up thinking that science is definite and concrete and scientists are sure and unbiased, and then we find that this is by no means the case and we are offered diametrically opposed views such as these.

So who can you trust? Well, you can trust people who have open minds; who don't pretend that they and their colleagues know everything about a disorder. This is true of cancer just as much as schizophrenia or depression. This doesn't mean they don't have a lot of experience which will allow you or your relative to be helped.

---

* Lidz, T. and Blatt, S. (1983). Critique of the Danish-American studies of the biological and adoptive relatives of adoptees who became schizophrenic. *American Journal of Psychiatry*, *140*, 426.

† Cassou, B., Schiff, M., and Stewart, J. (1980). Génétique et schizophrénie: Ré-évaluation d'un consensus. *Psychiatrie de l'Enfant*, *23*, 87.

It doesn't actually mean that schizophrenia is definitely not inherited – some sort of predisposition may well be inherited as may the types of small, subtle but important characteristics discussed in Chapter 11 – but this is still unproved. Basically there are no facts in schizophrenia, nor in most psychological disorders: there are ideas and opinions and hypotheses which are added to by our experience as helpers.

2) A biochemical cause?

For decades now there has been a search for a cause of schizophrenia which involves some change in the brain's chemistry. The determination to find such a source is hardly surprising, given that the disorder produces behaviours so different to other people's, and, in its chronic form may have such profound effects on the sufferer and those who are close. Moreover, the schizophrenic-type disorders are relatively common (one in a hundred suffer worldwide) and so are an enormous drain on financial and human resources, as well as creating immense human suffering. If the condition was caused by a chemical imbalance, it may not be so difficult to put it right.

Many theories of chemical imbalance have been tested over the years and all have been found wanting when stringent research methods have been applied. However, one theory which remains in favour and which has produced some good scientific research concerns possible changes in the levels of the neurotransmitters, dopamine and norepinephrine. Neurotransmitters are chemical messengers which carry the signal from one neurone (nerve cell) to the receptor sites of another. The theory suggests that too many of these neurotransmitters are produced in schizophrenic disorders, and it's the bombardment of the receptor sites with all these extra signals that causes the thought disorders and hallucinations.

This theory is supported by the fact that amphetamine, or 'speed' increases dopamine and norepinephrine levels, and amphetamine 'overdoses' have often been mistaken for schizophrenia when people come to hospital obviously psychotic. It may be then that the mind and body are reacting to too much dopamine and norepinephrine in schizophrenia in much the same way that they do with amphetamine. The other point that helps this argument is that the major tranquillisers, which have the effect of dampening down some of the symptoms, resemble the neuro-transmitters, and may therefore act by taking their place on the receptor sites and thereby blocking their effect. Of course, the fact that the drugs only reduce the intensity of the symptoms rather than produce 'normality' raises limitations about this part of the argument.

This theory is attractive, but only speculation: there's still no proof that the biochemistry of the brain actually changes in the ways suggested. Even if it does, this may be the product of some other underlying cause, whether physical or psychological. Certainly, other research suggests that stress has an effect on our biochemistry, so it may be that it is environmental conditions which change the levels of the neurotransmitters in some people, which in turn produce the unwanted behaviours.

The other main biochemical claims concern diet. A few clinicians (such as Mackarness) have argued that changing dietary patterns, perhaps by vitamin increase, or perhaps by testing for allergies, can result in cures for schizophrenia. Most of this work still rests on individual cases rather than large clinical trials, and is therefore not too convincing as yet: when we know that schizophrenia has so many problems in its diagnosis and many people who have psychotic breakdowns do not relapse, it's always possible that these cures took place on people who would have recovered on their own. So you should treat new 'miracle' cures with some healthy scepticism; however, in practice, with so much uncertainty concerning the disorder, it may seem worthwhile for you to try to tackle things on a number of fronts, including diet.

3) Is it society's fault?

Acute, short-lived psychotic breakdowns, with all the hallmarks of schizophrenic-type disorders, are quite common responses to severe stressors including a prolonged lack of sleep. Although they may be treated in the same way, with major tranquillisers, they often present none of the long-term problems of recurrence that we see in chronic disorders. The stress may be very obvious, much as occurred in 'shell-shock' in the first world war, or in some of the concentration camps during the second, or may be much less obvious, as occurs when you change cultures. Patrick describes this:

I'd just come back from two years in New Guinea, taking longer than I should have doing the fieldwork for my PhD. I came back to a round of parties with old friends and also, of course, a lot of new faces. My relationship with my girlfriend had broken up by letter, but it had been a bit of a shock to see her suddenly with her new boyfriend and hear about their plans to marry. I didn't think I was minding, but I suppose I was. I think I must have got very tired, and things started to feel very unreal.

After the quiet of New Guinea, everything was so terribly noisy and everywhere felt violent. The news frightened me. It was the time of the Yorkshire Ripper and a murder had happened less than a mile away the week I'd arrived back. I started to feel women looking at me as if they thought it was me, and that I was evil. I don't know when friends realised that things were going haywire, but finally I threw a stool through the TV because I thought the Chief Constable, who was talking on and on, was saying he was going to come out and get me. I went into hospital then, and stayed about six weeks. I really don't properly understand what happened to me, but I've had no problems since at all.

It may be that in such a new and vastly different culture, all the things that used to provide us with rewards and with a structure to our life fall away and, if we are feeling emotionally and physically frail, we have little left to grip on to. At such a time the very real horrors of the outside world are more transparently clear and mingle with our own deep-seated terrifying fantasies (what Conrad called 'The Heart of Darkness'). This is, of course, speculation, but it made sense to Patrick. In Yorkshire at that time it was true that women had reached the stage where they really did regard each man as a potential Ripper: in his sensitised state it would not have been difficult to pick up such accusations and perhaps to connect them to his own anger at his ex-girlfriend. Even the wildest delusions can sometimes make sense if you listen to them and see where they might fit in the person's life. As Shakespeare wrote in Hamlet: 'Though this be madness, yet there is method in it.'

There are clear aspects of our world which, viewed with the fresh eyes of an adolescent, will appear like madness, but which we have come to see as normal: parents who clearly detest each other, but stay together for their children's sake; terrible famines that exist side by side with butter, grain and meat mountains; super-powers who can continue to stockpile nuclear weapons despite the fact that one planeload would be sufficient for the total anni-hilation of mankind; and so on. As a result a number of writers over the years have questioned who is psychotic: those of us who manage to live in society with relative ease, or those who are unable to do so. One of the most formidable ways that society exerts its influence, for good and for ill, is through the family, and this has been a source of theories about the causes of schizophrenia since Freud's time and beyond.

Of course, it's not possible to know for sure whether certain sorts of parents will produce children who will grow up to be diagnosed as schizophrenic. The accounts of childhood will usually come from the patients themselves and it's always possible that they're affected by their disorder. However, much of the work conducted by Ronald Laing, the British psychiatrist, and his colleagues in the sixties (the 'anti-psychiatry' movement), involved watching families together and listening to their conver-sations, and this led to a number of theories about the ways that family interactions could produce a 'schizophrenic' way of behav-ing. From these he concluded:

> *In over 100 cases where we have studied the actual circumstances around the social event when one person comes to be regarded as schizophrenic, it seems tô us that without exception the experience and behaviour that gets labelled schizophrenic is a special strategy that a person invents in order to live in an unliveable situation.*

He goes on to talk about the 'contradictory and paradoxical pressures and demands, pushes and pulls, both internally, from himself, and externally, from those around him'. This 'checkmate' is the 'double-bind' or 'can't win' position described by Gregory Bateson back in 1956. Briefly, this arises from interactions between the child and parent when two messages are conveyed, one usually verbally (for example, 'You look tired darling. I think you should get some sleep now') and one by gesture or expression (implying, for example, 'The very sight of you around makes me sick'). Certainly prolonged exposure to these double messages are likely to make a child feel very unsure of itself, but this may come out in a number of ways including depression and anger, and research with those diagnosed as schizophrenic offered little support that it actually produces the disorder.

More recently, Leff and his colleagues at the Institute of Psychiatry in London, have offered more substantial proof that, at least for some sufferers, family dynamics may play a part in keeping the disorder going. They found the families to be higher on 'expressed emotion', by which they meant more critical and more over-protective than other families. The importance of this is shown by the therapeutic work with young sufferers which either aims to change the pattern of relating, via family therapy, or to distance the person from his or her family. These interventions certainly have a beneficial effect in preventing relapse, and this suggests (though doesn't prove) that over-critical or over-protective attitudes may have been one factor in the initial breakdown.

Most people in the field would agree that we have no firm knowledge about what causes schizophrenia. If it's genetic, then it may be biochemical; but without sound evidence showing its inheritability, any biochemical changes which might come are just as likely to be a reaction to the long-term or short-term stresses from your environment as they are the sudden development of a 'disease'. By realising this, we can approach the treatment of schizophrenic-type disorders in wider ways than merely using drugs.

THE TREATMENT OF SCHIZOPHRENIC-TYPE DISORDERS

If you suffer a psychotic breakdown of any type, chances are that someone else will encourage you to seek help. Although everything about you may feel 'wrong' in schizophrenic-type disorders, there's little space left in your thinking to allow you to actually realise this. If you refuse help you may well be hospitalised compulsorily (or 'sectioned') for a time under the Mental Health Act (see p. 19).

Whether you are treated in hospital or at home (more usual in second and subsequent bouts), you will almost inevitably be given one of the major tranquillising drugs, such as Largactil (chlorpromazine) or Haldol (haloperidol). As the more extreme of your behaviours reduce, the dose will be lowered and, if this is your first breakdown and especially if it seemed to be a reaction to something stressful, it will finally be stopped. If things get bad again shortly after you stop the drugs, then you may be advised to continue taking some form of the drug for a much longer period, perhaps by way of long-acting injections such as Modecate.

The principal helpful effect of these drugs is in reducing the feelings of panic and desperation and taking away some of the most agitated frightened behaviour. Lena described the effects as 'turning down the volume control on all that's happening'. After a series of breakdowns from the age of 19, she has since married and had a family and works as a nurse. She has occasionally tried stopping the drugs, both because she felt OK and because she suffered some of the less severe side-effects, but relapsed quickly. In this more chronic form of the disorder, around half of the sufferers relapse when they stop their drugs – but of course, this means that about half stay OK without them. If you've been on major tranquillisers for many years you and your doctor may feel that it's worth the risk, every few years, to see how well you manage without them.

Although the drugs aren't addictive, they can have some very distressing or even dangerous side-effects, so clearly they should never be used unnecessarily. The most serious side-effects are rare – for example, hepatitis (liver inflammation) and hyperpyrexia (raised body temperature which can lead to heatstroke and even death) – but tardive dyskinesias (writhing muscle movements, usually of the neck up, which are very disfiguring and often permanent) occur in quite a large proportion of people if they take the drugs for a number of years.

Almost everyone taking the drugs will feel drowsy for the first few days, and have a dry mouth for several weeks. You may also find yourself dizzy when you stand up quickly, and constipation is often a problem. In addition there are a number of muscular problems that you might suffer initially, such as feelings of cramp in your neck and mouth. If this happens tell your doctor, because they can quickly be stopped by other medication. You may also feel that you can't sit still, but have to keep walking up and down or fidgeting, and you'll often experience trembling. Another frightening side-effect is an enormous feeling of stiffness in your face or legs or arms. Ginny described this to me:

The first time I took the drugs I was really psychotic and the experience of taking them was hard to unscramble from everything else that seemed to be happening to me. I had a horrific three days of muscular spasms where nothing seemed to move right, and yet no one seemed to notice. I didn't really appreciate that these were drug effects rather than me being mad until the second time I was given them. Then I wasn't psychotic but had just started to speed up and be anxious. I was coming back from the launderette and found I simply couldn't walk properly. I couldn't bend my knees at all and it was so embarrassing. It took me ten minutes to get five yards because my mind and body seemed so separated.

This time I knew clearly that this was because of the drugs, but I think a lot of people won't be articulating their experiences – they'll look back on them as just part of the psychosis, and they're not. For example, one man told me he felt as though someone was pulling fingernails down a blackboard, but right through his body. I'd felt this too, and it was so useful to have someone else put it into words and to realise it was the drugs. They don't tell you what to expect in hospital, and so you don't know what's normal side-effects and what's part of being psychotic.

These drugs do allow many people to operate much more normally within society. However, because of their potency and the severity of some of their side-effects they should *never* be taken unless absolutely necessary and always with expert advice, and their use should be regularly reviewed.

Psychotherapy

Psychotherapy is used less frequently for psychotic breakdowns in this country than in the States where it's often used in the private sphere. This is not surprising since anyone who advocates it usually emphasises the length of time required to bring about change. Drugs are obviously much speedier and, in the long run, much less expensive, and so psychotherapy is rarely offered, especially to chronic sufferers. However, as Patrick's story shows (p. 198), many delusions and hallucinations can be understood if you care to look for meaning.

An article by Angela Douglas* described a woman who was

* Douglas, A. (1986). Psychotherapy in institutional settings: Another look. *Changes*, 4, 158.

psychotic and in a seclusion cell for her own protection. She was incontinent, had lost most of her words and, if let out, jumped on other patients and stole from them. In their first meeting she spoke two sentences: 'Both my parents are dead,' and 'I cook and I clean at home, that's all I do.' This and other parts of her behaviour revealed both a desperately bewildered little child and a realistically distressed adult, and the ward staff treated her accordingly. She was given a proper room of her own with her own things and the nurses cared for her lovingly, like a baby, while a doctor took time to talk to her and encourage her adult part. Within a week she was continent, dressing herself, and eating and mixing with other patients. She started to structure her 'care plan' according to her own wishes, with the reassurance and encouragement of her nurses.

Although she was not given a diagnosis of schizophrenia, the case shows that a psychotherapeutic approach may be possible even in severe psychotic breakdowns and may have more long-term effects than medication. However, good well-designed research of effectiveness is difficult and very expensive, especially when therapy may take years, and so far there has been little evidence accumulated to show real change. Nevertheless, many case studies make it clear that the possibility for change does exist through psychotherapy, which suggests not that the door is boarded up but that we have not yet found the right key for everyone. The problem is that while these disorders are thought of as illnesses to be cured only by drugs, then money is simply not going to be allocated towards the proper training in and evaluation of a psychotherapeutic approach. Pharmaceutical companies are some of the richest in the world and can afford the very expensive research involved in showing the effectiveness of drugs.

Changing the environment

Research shows that urban areas have somewhat higher rates for schizophrenic-type disorders than rural ones and this line of thinking has been followed by some organisations in providing safe, calm therapeutic societies for people to live in. Johnny became clearly withdrawn when he was 16. He began muttering to himself and staying in his room and, if you insisted, he would tell you about the chemical warhead that was kept in the loft.

Rather than diagnosing him as schizophrenic, the psychiatrist managed to have him taken into one of the Rudolph Steiner country homes where he learnt farming and living in a caring community and did well.

The work that takes place in therapeutic communities also shows that you can certainly recover from *acute* disorders without drugs just as well as you can with them; although perhaps more slow, recovery may be longer-lasting. It's certainly true that some people will always find it difficult to live in our speedy violent society, but perhaps we should take that as our problem rather than theirs and provide more of these alternatives.

Changing the environment is the aim of family therapy and Leff's work (p. 201) has shown that using this method to allow the parents to be less critical and less protective of the young man or woman has beneficial effects in preventing relapse. In families who will not attend for family therapy or who do not manage to change sufficiently, providing somewhere in the community away from the family home also helps to prevent another episode occurring. This is not to say that all families need family therapy: only that it is a useful approach in those who show the pattern of being over-critical and over-protective.

Help for families

Living with someone who has a schizophrenic-type disorder is certainly very difficult, whether you are their parent, sibling or child. The National Schizophrenia Fellowship provides help and information for both sufferers and relatives. However, it does take a clear illness model of the disorder. It has a range of publications and has set up hostels, sheltered workshops and drop-in centres. The Richmond Fellowship has similar facilities and your local MIND will also provide information and may put you in touch with other people in your position. Gaining as much knowledge as you can, talking to others with similar problems, and becoming involved in the politics of providing good services are all seen as good ways of coping.

PARANOID DISORDERS

Being a little paranoic – not totally trusting people, being a little sceptical or cynical – seems quite useful in a world that has its share of acquisitiveness and violence. However, if this colours the way that you approach everything, chances are you will have fewer friends and you will miss the joys of life to such an extent that it may be seen as a psychological problem. Clinical work has shown these people often have a perfectionist parent sensitive to what people think; they've often been labelled as unique in some way when young (very good-looking, talented, etc.), and may have suffered bullying at school. Chances are, if you recognise yourself in this you will probably also be pretty isolated, especially from the opposite sex, and will spend a lot of time wondering why.

Such a problem is only a mild extension of normal scepticism and certainly not an illness. But if it's making your life less full and if you're lonely you may consider seeking help. A cognitive-behaviour therapist might look at your fears of being evaluated socially and teach you anxiety management and social skills so you don't feel you 'stand out'. Psychodynamic psychotherapy might look at your problems in trusting the therapist and others and the ways these relate to early experiences.

At the extreme, people can become so totally suspicious that they do become psychotic, believing 'They' are trying to get them in ways far beyond the possibilities of reality. If these people are still able to function all right, then they may still simply be labelled as eccentric; if not they may be hospitalised and given major tranquillisers.

Paranoid psychosis can occur without any additional problems, or as part of the manic phase of manic-depression (Chapter 14), in some depressive disorders, or in a paranoid form of a schizophrenic psychosis, probably as the result of a particular hallucination or delusion. Even at this extreme, it's often possible to make sense of this in terms of the person's life; for example, old people (see Chapter 12, p. 179) may become severely paranoid but this often begins with realistic fears of violence and theft, or battles with relatives or the Social Security, or simply because they are becoming deaf.

As Roy Porter describes in *A Social History of Madness,** many of
the fears and irrational beliefs of peoples in different times and
situations, if really listened to, appear much more understandable
when we hear them within the context of society and its current
pressures.

---

* 'A Social History of Madness – Stories of the Insane,' by Roy Porter,
Weidenfeld & Nicolson, 1987.

Chapter

Mania and manic-depression

In 1962, at the age of 25, John Ogdon's genius as a pianist was recognised when he was awarded the prize at the Moscow International Tchaikovsky Competition, sharing it with the legendary Ashkenazy. His fame was quickly established around the world and success continued until, in the early seventies, he began suffering from frightening changes in mood. In an article in *The Sunday Times* (21.6.81) entitled 'Madly Gifted', his wife described his breakdown as she saw it.

It seemed to begin with a gradual obsession with a charity organiser who had hurt his feelings by questioning his generosity. Over the next few months he began to show an 'apparent determination to shock' which alternated with his old character of absent-minded genius. He would suddenly become very irritable and fly into rages in which she sometimes feared for her life. Occasionally he would let her know that he needed help, but when it arrived it was usually refused. Interspersed between the abnormal behaviour and the man she knew were three serious suicide attempts and self-mutilation. John Ogdon was eventually diagnosed as suffering from manic-depression.

Whereas depression is a lowering of your mood with sadness, low self-esteem and often a slowing down of all effort and activity, in mania your mood turns towards elation, you begin to feel you could do anything and your activity increases to such an extent that collapsing from physical exhaustion becomes a real risk.

Mania and manic-depression

Mania is classed as a psychotic disorder, not just because of your abnormal behaviour (although it's usually very bizarre, initially it is rather more on a continuum with normal behaviour than is a schizophrenic-type disorder), but also because you rarely have any insight into the fact that things are going badly out of control. Many of the problems concerning diagnosis and labelling that were discussed in the last chapter apply also to mania and manic-depression.

Hypomania is the term used for less severe forms of the disorder where you're likely to feel very 'high' or euphoric, where you talk incessantly and rush round doing things, and where your friends and relatives might notice that you're coming out with some unusually shocking remarks. Doreen is a senior nurse in a large teaching hospital:

I'd got very run down. There were dreadful staff shortages and I'd been working far too hard, not taking any breaks and worrying constantly about things. It wasn't irrational worrying: you know that eventually with people trying to cope under so much pressure, something's going to go wrong, and on a ward like ours that can be fatal. I started to feel more and more unreal; it sometimes felt as if my feet weren't quite touching the ground. I remember wondering on one or two occasions if I could fly. It seemed to let me do everything even faster. I was starting to enjoy the sensation of speeding along. I wasn't sleeping much; just an hour or two a night. The rest of the time I'd plan new rotas or talk to anyone else around. I talked and talked.

I know I came out with quite a few risque remarks. I can't really remember what they were but I can remember the expressions on people's faces as I'd let something slip. Finally I made some comment on my sex life in the middle of a ward-round, and the consultant took me into his office and called a psychiatrist and they both decided it was time I had a break. I couldn't see that there was anything wrong at all and so refused to take the drugs they offered. Eventually they had to have me sectioned in order to get me into hospital and get some drugs into me. Actually, it wasn't awful. I felt more amused than distressed that they couldn't understand that I was fine. I stayed in hospital a couple of weeks and I think I spent most of it asleep: I really needed that. I've been fine ever since.

During more severe manias, the feelings that you can do anything and that you have enormous energy may lead to some very extraordinary behaviour. Jason was a headmaster. He had had a series of huge mood swings during the week before he was admitted to hospital, switching from being very high and expansive to feeling desperately depressed, and with brief periods of the normal him in-between. His wife and doctor had managed to persuade him to go into hospital during one of these times when he was able to realise that things were out of control. However, he slipped out of the ward very shortly after his admission and went into town. He spent £5,000 in an hour and then travelled first-class down to London. He booked into the Dorchester and began to organise an international conference on teaching methods, hiring 50 temporary secretaries, a conference centre, ordering reams of embossed letterheaded paper and making dozens of long international phone-calls. In the two days before they found him, he had run up bills and contracts for thousands and thousands of pounds.

This enormous expansiveness and generosity can obviously cause domestic tragedy and financial ruin. In Jason's case, most of it could be returned to normal, but other men and women have given away their house, auctioned off their Aston Martin, and handed over their unemployment benefit the moment it was in their hands. Instead of buying one packet of cigarettes, they buy two dozen; rather than buy a small round of drinks, they treat the whole pub. Like Jason, they may have wonderful schemes for changing the world and usually consider themselves to have all the necessary powers to bring this about. In addition to delusions like this, they may also have both visual and auditory hallucinations, and at this point it will be very difficult for psychiatrists to decide whether they should be diagnosed as having a schizophrenic-type disorder or one involving mania.

In the early stages, people report that the elation is pleasant and others certainly enjoy having them around, whereas in schizophrenia you really don't feel good at all and life feels overwhelming rather than letting you feel you could do anything. However, as things get more out of control in mania, the state of excitement becomes less pleasant. Unlike schizophrenia, if manic disorders do come again they tend to come just in episodes, letting people operate fairly normally in-between. These episodes may be years apart or may recur more and more frequently leaving little time between them.

Despite the almost endearing qualities of early mania, mood swings can make people generous and laughing one moment, and irritable or even raging and violent the next. If you are suffering from this disorder anything more than mildly, chances are you will be admitted to hospital for both your own safety and sometimes for that of others.

Except in mild cases of hypomania, the cheerful expansive mood rarely continues uninterrupted, which is why the term 'manic-depression' is used more often than mania. Nurses who attend sufferers throughout the whole day and night report that, in many of them, their mood changes very frequently: the higher they are one minute the more desperately depressed they are the next. These periods of depression can last from minutes to hours, and in longer ones the risk of suicide is very real. Sophie, a dentist, had had some sort of breakdown ten years earlier when she was in her twenties: she remembered feeling very 'speedy' and doing ten things at once but had had no problems since. Now she was married and she and her husband had recently bought their first house together. Her husband remembered that she'd been in a particularly good mood for the last few days and presumed she was simply very excited about the new house. As he said:

> *She hardly seemed to need any sleep, and one morning she brought me a cup of tea at about six o'clock and stayed chatting for a couple of hours, describing her plans to turn the back garden into a tennis court and swimming-pool combined. I was aware on one level that this was crazy, but everyone says crazy things sometimes. She stopped talking quite abruptly and left the room and minutes later I heard her drive off— to work, I thought. But she accelerated the car to about 60 miles per hour and drove very accurately into the supports of the railway bridge. Remarkably she survived with only a broken wrist.*

So it is important that help is sought: you simply can't rely on the person concerned to know that something is going wrong. When mood changes in the way it does in manic-depressive disorders, there are often times in-between the extremes where the person is their old self once again and those close are often swift in presuming that everything is going to be all right. John Ogdon's wife put the problem like this:

My failure to realise what was happening is not explicable in terms of society and background alone; in matters of the unbalanced brain it is, I believe, a sad paradox that it is often our love for the victim that blinds us to his true condition. Quite simply, it is virtually impossible to grasp that someone we are very close to – someone to whom we talk every day, someone we sleep with, and play with, and work with, and who is an integral part of our very existence – it is impossible to conceive or to grasp that this person may be going out of his mind.

THE CAUSES OF MANIC-DEPRESSION

Except in the most severe cases, manic-depression does not carry with it the sense of a life-sentence that a diagnosis of schizophrenia will often imply. Although bouts of the disorder may continue all through your life, the gaps in-between can be very long and you can operate perfectly normally at those times. Many psychiatrists regard the mood swings as difficult to explain in ways other than biochemical, but no chemical factor has been found to account for the change.

The same arguments that were discussed in the chapter on schizophrenia apply equally to manic-depression. Even if it's the case that the condition is caused immediately by a change in brain chemistry, this does not rule out the fact that this change is likely to have been brought about by some external cause – perhaps by prolonged stress, as happened to Doreen, or by a change in circumstances, such as Sophie's marriage and what that might have meant to her. Certainly most of the research shows that a large proportion of people suffering their first bout of mania have had a clear life event during the month before it began.

Quite often people will approach grief, such as the death of a spouse, by a period of manic activity which allows them to be 'too busy to think'. When they finally stop, grief rushes in – painful but necessary.

The same pattern of mania and depression may operate on a more permanent scale as one strategy of trying to block out the anger and pain of a wretched childhood. Psychological approaches have suggested that various family relations might predispose you to manic-depression. For example, one psychoanalytic study suggested that these families, more than most, try to improve their status and are more envious and competitive. The person with the disorder has had to carry the rest of the family's ambitions and so feels it necessary to strive extra hard and feels guilty at any set-backs. It's quite likely that a family background like this would produce some kind of psychological problem, though not necessarily manic-depression.

Just as with schizophrenia, there have been a number of studies conducted in order to try to discover whether manic-depression, or at least something which predisposes us to the disorder, could be inherited. These concluded that, while there was no evidence that depression alone was inherited, there was quite strong evidence that there was some genetic ingredient involved in a proportion of manic-depression cases. The studies have not received the same critical scrutiny as those did which looked at the schizophrenia research, but it's quite possible that the same statistical problems exist to throw doubt on how much we can rely on their conclusions. In David Wigoder's excellent account of his manic-depression, *Images of Destruction*, the foreword by Storr stresses the genetic argument by pointing to the insane behaviour of Wigoder's mother. In fact her awful behaviour could be quite sufficient to explain her son's pattern of achievement and destruction without adding some imaginary genetic factor.

THE TREATMENT OF MANIC-DEPRESSIVE DISORDERS

It's acknowledged in many psychiatric textbooks that mild bouts of mania may come and go without any treatment; by some means the person is able to work his or her way through the psychosis and out the other side. Sometimes they will recognise later that things were definitely becoming rather peculiar for them, and sometimes they won't. However, once you start spending vast sums of money, or getting into fights, or laying elaborate plans to cure the world of some particular ill, continuing endlessly day and night, then it's likely that someone close to you, or your GP, or the police will make sure you get psychiatric help.

Tim kept his wife awake half the night talking endlessly about his views on life and his reasons for not believing himself to be mad; he visited his GP several times a day with a similar agenda.

In such a situation, it's quite likely that tolerance runs out and everyone agrees that drugs, and possibly hospitalisation, are required. And it's not just a question of other people's tolerance: your body simply can't go on and on without rest in the way your mind thinks it can, and, without help, people may exhaust themselves to the point of collapse.

The drugs most commonly given when hypomania or manic-depression is first diagnosed are the major tranquillisers, such as Largactil (chlorpromazine) and Serenace or Haldol (haloperidol). Because it's so difficult for patients to understand that they have a problem, and are causing a problem to others, these drugs may be given in quite strong doses initially, and sometimes by injection instead of tablet form. In addition to the side-effects discussed on p. 202, a stronger dose often produces others, such as tremor or muscular problems in the eyes and neck. The drugs will be gradually reduced to a level that still controls the behaviour and will probably be continued for several weeks if all seems well.

This will be the pattern of treatment for the first two or three bouts of a manic-depressive disorder. At that time it will probably be suggested that you begin to take lithium carbonate. This is generally accepted by the medical profession to be the most effective preventative drug treatment for manic-depression, reducing both the mania and the depression. The reason that it's not given at the first diagnosis is that, once again, the side-effects can be severe and so it's not thought worth the risk involved if the psychosis was going to be a single unrepeated event – which many are.

When you first take lithium you will need blood tests taken every few days so that plasma levels can be monitored; once the right dose for you has been found, you'll probably need a test once a month or even less. If the levels are right, lithium is not an uncomfortable drug to take, though some people dislike the flatness of mood that it produces. However, if the levels are wrong it can prove extremely dangerous. Early signs of problems are a marked tremor in your hands and slight nausea or discomfort around your stomach area. More serious are drowsiness, vomiting and diarrhoea: for any of these signs you must contact your doctor immediately. If you find yourself getting up four or five times a night to pass urine, you should also consult your doctor. You probably won't be given lithium if you have any history of heart or kidney problems.

Because lithium actually seems to prevent attacks of manic-depression, the only way to know whether you still need it is to stop it and see. Of course, you should always consult your doctor about this, but some psychiatrists suggest that you might try stopping every two years or so.

Like all the drugs that are prescribed for psychological disorders, lithium does not cure the disorder, but it may give you space in which to learn to discover more about what's causing the problem – whether these forces are external, in the way of stress, or internal in the way of psychological conflicts. Whereas psychotherapy is very commonly given for depression, for mania or manic-depression, as in all psychoses, it's very rarely offered. However, Wigoder's book, *Images of Destruction*, is an account of his own group and individual therapy provided by the NHS, which he clearly found very valuable. In other countries, for example Israel and the States, therapy is used more, often alongside drug treatment.

In a recent article on psychotherapy for mania, Roberto Mester* described Renan, a young man who had been conscripted into the army. After two weeks he refused to obey his officers and gradually became more and more tense and excited and gave orders, stating he was the commander. He tore around everywhere and talked non-stop, often declaring that he could cure everyone in the world. Sometimes he would tell people he was a doctor, and he clearly had an ambition to study medicine. He was placed on major tranquillisers to calm him and, as they were being reduced, he started psychotherapy. His therapist learnt how his father had died of a sudden heart attack in front of Renan when he was nine. No one in the family would talk about it, but it had triggered a dream in Renan to become a cardiologist – helping to cure what he'd once 'allowed' to happen. He had hoped to be on a medical unit in the army, but this was refused, and the frustration this caused to such a long and deeply held ambition was thought to be an important factor in his mania. Talking about his father's death at last, and also about the strength of his ambition and what it meant to him, seemed to relieve his symptoms and so the drugs were stopped. He was still fine 12 months later.

* Mester, R. (1986). The psychotherapy of mania. *British Journal of Medical Psychology*, *59*, 13.

215

Mania is so distressing and potentially so dangerous that it can very rarely be left untreated by drugs, and perhaps they will always be necessary initially, even if just to stop the person dying from exhaustion. But, as in all psychological problems, the use of drugs should never stop any of us – professionals, sufferers and those close to them – looking for or fighting for additional and alternative forms of help. Becoming involved in the politics of the mental health services, perhaps through the organisation MIND, will be an important way of keeping abreast of the issues and pressing for the funding and evaluation of other forms of treatment.

Appendix:
Relaxation

This relaxation takes 12–15 minutes, or longer if you wish. It is based on an 'autogenic training' method and aims to help you to become more and more aware of your body. This process allows you to recognise when parts of your body are becoming tense and when they are relaxed. It's best practised sitting in a comfortable chair somewhere fairly peaceful. Take the phone of the hook, but don't worry about everyday noise of traffic, chatter, etc. I prefer to have my hands in my lap touching each other, and it's better to place both feet on the floor. The 'awareness' that's talked about isn't gained by moving the parts of your body, but by directing your attention to that part. If possible read the following on to a tape, pausing at the dots, or get someone to read it out slowly to you. In the silence you can use the word 'Relax' as suggested (or any other word you want: some people simply say 'one') or visualise a warm pleasant scene – whatever suits you best.

sitting comfortably . . . and becoming aware of all the feelings and sensations in your body . . . thinking first of your hands . . . and recognising the surfaces where they touch each other and where they touch your clothes . . . and becoming aware of any feelings within your hands . . . any warmth or coolness . . . any numbness or tingling . . . just become aware of the feelings in your hands . . . and let them become warm and comfortable and relaxed. . . . Thinking now of your arms . . . recognising the surfaces where they touch your clothes and your body . . . and becoming aware of any feelings within them . . . any warmth, any tingling, any heaviness . . . any tension in your arms, recognise it and let it go . . . just let it go . . . replaced by relaxation . . . your arms becoming warm and comfortable and relaxed. . . . Now think about your feet . . . the surfaces inside your shoes, resting on the floor . . . and become aware of any feelings within your feet . . . any warmth or coolness, any numbness or tingling . . . just become aware of the feelings within your feet, and let them become warm, and comfortable and relaxed. . . . Think about your legs . . . recognise the surfaces where they touch your clothes . . . where they press into the chair . . . and any feelings within your legs . . . any tingling, any coolness . . . any heaviness . . . any tension in your legs . . . recognise it . . . and let it go . . . just let it go . . . replaced by relaxation . . . your legs becoming warm, comfortable and relaxed. . . . Think about your shoulders . . . and your back . . . recognise the surfaces where they touch your clothes, where they touch the chair . . . recognise any tension around your neck, your shoulders, . . . recognise it, and let it go . . . just let it go . . . replaced by relaxation . . . your shoulders heavy, relaxed and comfortable. . . . Now think about your face . . . recognise any feelings on the surface of your face, any coolness, warmth . . . and any feelings within . . . any tingling, any coolness . . . recognise the gentle weight of your cheeks . . . of your jaw, your tongue . . . now just let your face become smooth, relaxed, comfortable. . . . Think about your stomach . . . recognise it as it rises and falls, with each breath, in and out . . . any tension in your stomach . . . recognise it and let it go . . . just let it go . . . replaced by relaxation . . . your stomach warm, comfortable and relaxed. . . . Now think about your breathing . . . recognise the breath, as it goes in and out . . . and in and out . . . of your body. . . . And with each breath out . . . the tension leaves your body . . . tension leaves your body with each breath out. . . . Your whole body now . . . comfortable, and relaxed . . . and as you sit there, just say the word relax to yourself . . . just lightly, like a thought . . . just let it flicker through your mind . . . relax . . . relax . . . (leave silence of 3 minutes here). . . . *Checking your body again for spots of tension . . . and letting it go. . . . I'm going to count back from 6 to 1 and at 1 your feelings of heaviness will go and you'll be refreshed. 6–5–4 . . . lighter and lighter 3–2–1.*(End)

This is not hypnosis, but the last part is just for safety for the one or two who may go into a really deep relaxation.

Like all skills, relaxation needs practice – hopefully twice a day for the first few weeks. It's best done on an empty stomach. Use the tape as much as you wish at the beginning and then do it from memory wherever you want – at work, in the train, in bed, standing in the supermarket – wherever you feel tense or anxious. It won't pull you out of a really high state of anxiety or panic but it will work for general tension and will gradually teach you to recognise early when your tension is building up so you can do a relaxation and prevent anxiety taking over. How long it takes you to reach this useful stage varies with each individual – from days to months – but *everyone* benefits from it eventually, both physically and psychologically. So keep it up.

Further Information:
Books and Organisations

CHAPTER 2

Useful Books

A Place Like This: A Guide to Life in a Psychiatric Hospital by R. Grainger, Churchman, 1984.

Behaviour Can Change by E. V. S. Westmacott and R. J. Cameron, Macmillan, 1981.

Families and How to Survive Them by Robin Skynner and John Cleese, Methuen, 1983.

Images of Destruction by D. Wigoder, Routledge and Kegan Paul, 1987.

Mental Illness and the Law by T. Whitehead, Blackwell, 1983.

Psychiatry for Beginners by Eia Asen, Unwin, 1986.

Taking Care: An Alternative to Therapy by David Smail, Dent, 1987.

Talking to a Stranger: A Consumer's Guide by Lindsay Knight, Penguin Books, 1986.

Voices – Psychoanalysis edited by B. Bourne, Spokesman Press, 1987.

The Words to Say It by Marie Cardinal, Picador, 1983.

Organisations

MIND 22 Harley Street, London WIN 2ED (071–637 0741; or in your local phone directory).

MIND Yourself Project and MIND Bookshop 155/157 Woodhouse Lane, Leeds LS2 3ED (0532 430918).

Richmond Fellowship 8 Addison Road, London W14 8DL (071–603 6373).

Self-Help Team 114 Mansfield Road, Nottingham NG1 3HL (0602 691212).

Australian National Association of the Mental Health 1 Cookson Street, Campberwell, VIC 3141, Australia ((03) 813 1180).

CHAPTER 3

Useful Books

Bereavement – Studies of Grief in Adult Life by C. M. Parkes, Penguin Books, 1986.

Calm Down – How to Cope with Frustration and Anger by P. Hanck, Sheldon Press, 1984.

Coping With Stress: A Guide to Living Wiley Self-Teaching Guides, Wiley, 1982.

Coping with Crises by Glenys Parry, British Psychological Society and Routledge 1990.

Stress Check by C. L. Cooper, Spectrum, 1983.

On Unemployment

The Healing Echo by E. Heimler, Souvenir Press, 1986.

Hope on the Dole by T. Walter, SPCK, 1985.

Organisations

Cruse Cruse House 126 Sheen Road, Richmond TW9 1UR (081–940 4818; or in your local phone directory).

Stress Control Centre 5 Victoria Parade, Manly, NSW 2095, Australia ((02) 977 5200).

National Association for Loss & Grief 35 Kedumba Crescent, Turramurra, NSW 2074, Australia ((02) 988 3376).

CHAPTER 4

Useful Books

See the books on 'stress' for Chapter 3.

Coming Off Tranquillisers and Sleeping Pills by Shirley Trickett, Thorsons, 1986.

Illusions and Reality: The Meaning of Anxiety by David Smail, Dent, 1984.

Ok2 Talk Feelings by Jenny Cozens, BBC Books, 1991.

'That's Life!' Survey on Tranquillisers by R. Lacey and S. Woodward, BBC/MIND, 1985.

Organisations

Council for Involuntary Tranquilliser Addiction (CITA) Cavendish House, Brighton Road, Waterloo, Liverpool L22 5NG (Helpline 051 940 102).

CHAPTER 5

Useful Books

See 'stress' books for Chapter 3.

Agoraphobia by R. H. Vose, Faber and Faber, 1986.

Agoraphobia: Simple Effective Treatment by C. Weeks, Angus and Robertson, 1977.

Organisations

The Phobics Society 4 Cheltenham Road, Chorlton-cum-Hardy, Manchester M21 1QN (061 881 1937).

CHAPTER 6

Useful Books

Change for the Better by Elizabeth Wilde McCormick, Unwin Paperbacks, 1990.

Dealing with Depression by K. Nairne and G. Smith, Women's Press, 1984.

Depression: The Way Out of Your Prison by D. Rowe, Routledge and Kegan Paul, 1984.

Images of Destruction by D. Wigoder, Routledge and Kegan Paul, 1987.

The Pursuit of Happiness by P. Watzlawick, Norton, 1984.

The Savage God by A. Alvarez, Penguin Books, 1974.

Organisations

Depressives Associated PO Box 5, Castletowen, Portland, Dorset DT5 1BQ.

The Homestart Consultancy 2 Salisbury Road, Leicester LE1 7QR (0533 554988).

Newpin Sutherland House, Sutherland Square, Walworth, London SE17 (071–703 5271).

Samaritans 46 Marshall Street, London W1 (071–734 2800).

CHAPTER 7

Useful Books

Beat PMT Through Diet by M. Stewart, Ebury Press, 1987.

Depression After Childbirth by K. Dalton, Oxford University Press, 1980.

Female Cycles by P. Weideger, Women's Press, 1978.

The Loneliness of the Dying by N. Elias, Blackwell, 1985.

Menopause: A Positive Approach by R. Reitz, Unwin, 1981.

The Pre-Menstrual Syndrome and Progesterone Therapy by K. Dalton, Heinemann Medical, 1984.

Postnatal Depression by V. Welburn, Fontana, 1980.

Organisations

Association for Post-Natal Illness Institute of Obstetrics and Gynaecology, Queen Charlotte's Maternity Hospital, 399 Goldhawk Road, Hammersmith, London W6 0XG (071–748 4666).

British Colostomy Association 15 Station Road, Reading, Berks RG1 1LG (0734 391537).

Cancer Link 17 Britannia Street, London WC1X 9JN (071–833 2451).

The Homestart Consultancy 2 Salisbury Road, Leicester LE1 7QR (0533 554988).

Mastectomy Association of Great Britain 15–19 Britten Street, London SW3 3TZ (071–837 0908).

ME Association PO Box 8, Stanford-le-Hope, Essex SS17 8EX.

Newpin Sutherland House, Sutherland Square, Walworth, London SE17 (071–703 5271).

Women's Therapy Centre 6 Manor Gardens, London N7 6LA (071–263 6200).

CHAPTER 8

Useful Books

See the 'stress' books for Chapter 3.

CHAPTER 9

Useful Books

The Anorexic Experience by M. Lawrence, The Women's Press, 1984.
Coping with Bulimia by B. French, Thorsons, 1987.
Fat is a Feminist Issue by S. Orbach, Hamlyn, 1979.
Fed Up and Hungry Edited by M. Lawrence, The Women's Press, 1987.

Organisations

Anorexic Aid (also for Bulimia) The Priory Centre, 11 Priory Road, High Wycombe HP13 6SL (0494 521431).
Women's Therapy Centre 6 Manor Gardens, London N7 6LA (01–263 6200).

CHAPTER 10

Useful Books

Alcohol

Alcohol: Our Favourite Drug Royal College of Psychiatrists, 1986.
Coming Off Drink by J. and J. Ditzler, Papermac, 1987.
Codependency: How to Break free and Live Your Own Life by David Stafford and Liz Hodgkinson, Piatkus Books, 1991.
The Courage to Change: Personal Conversations About Alcoholism by D. Wholey, Fontana, 1984.
Of Course You're Anxious by Gayle Rosellini and Mark Worden, Hazleden Press, 1990.
Let's Drink to Your Health by I. Robertson and N. Heather, British Psychological Society, 1986.

Women Who Love Too Much by R. Norwood, Arrow Books, 1986.

Drugs
Drug Problems – Where to Get Help BBC, 1986.
Living with Drugs by M. Gossop, Wildwood House, 1987.

Organisations

Alcohol
The *ACCEPT* Clinic 724 Fulham Road, London sw6 5SE (071–371 7477).
AlAnon Family Groups (for the family and friends of problem drinkers) 61 Great Dover Street, London SE1 4YF (071–403 0888).
Alcoholics Anonymous PO Box 1, Stonebow House, Stonebow, York YO1 2NJ (0904 644026).
Alcoholics Anonymous 127 Edwin Street, Croydon, NSW 2132, Australia ((02) 799 1199).

Drugs
Drug Treatment Centre (help and advice for young people) 53 Basement, Vincent Square, London sw1.
Families Anonymous (for relatives and friends) 650 Holloway Road, London w19 3NU (071–281 8889).
Directorate of the Drug Offensive Level 7, 73 Miller Street, North Sydney, NSW 2060, Australia ((02) 391 9000).

Gambling
Gamblers Anonymous (information also on GamAnon Family Groups and Young GA) PO Box 88, London sw10 0EU (081–741 4181).
Gamblers Anonymous 53 Regent Street, Sydney, NSW 2000, Australia ((02) 951 555).

CHAPTER 11

Useful Books

Behaviour Can Change by E. V. S. Westmacott and R. J. Cameron, Macmillan, 1981.

Coping Successfully With Your Hyperactive Child by P. Carson, Sheldon, 1987.

Dibs in Search of Self by V. Axeline, Penguin Books, 1964.

Drugwatch: Just Say No by S. Caplin and S. Woodward, Corgi, 1986.

Drug Problems: Where to Get Help BBC, 1986.

Families and How to Survive Them by R. Skynner and J. Cleese, Methuen, 1983.

For Your Own Good: The Roots of Violence in Child-Rearing by A. Miller, Virago, 1987.

Help Your Child Cope with Stress by B. Remsburg and A. Saunders, Piatkus Books, 1985.

Living with A Teenager by S. Hayman, Piatkus Books, 1988.

My Problem Child by Nick Yapp, Penguin, 1991.

Living With Teenagers by M. Herbert, Blackwell, 1987.

Psychology and Parenthood by Jean Gross, Open University Press, 1989.

Women Who Love Too Much by R. Norwood, Arrow Books, 1986.

Organisations

Brook Advisory Centres 153a East Street, London SE17 2SD (071–708 1234).

Compassionate Friends 6 Denmark Street, Bristol BS1 5DQ (0272 292778).

Drug Treatment Centre (help and advice for young people) 53 Basement, Vincent Square, London SW1.

Families Anonymous (for families and friends) 650 Holloway Road, London N19 3NU (071–281 8889).

Hyperactive Children's Support Group 71 Whyke Lane, Chichester, West Sussex PO19 2LD (0903 725182).

Brandon Centre 26 Prince of Wales Road, London NW5 3LG (071–267 4792).

NSPCC 67 Saffron Hill, London EC1N 8RS (071–242 1626).

Samaritans See your local directory.

Tavistock Clinic 120 Belsize Lane, London NW3 5BA (071–435 7111).

CHAPTER 12

Useful Books

Alzheimer's Disease: A Guide for Families by L. S. Powell and K. Couttice, Addison-Wesley, 1983.

Bereavement – Studies of Grief in Adult Life by C. M. Parkes, Penguin Books, 1986.

Cure for the Elderly by J. Willingha, Optima, 1987.

The Caring Trap by J. Pulling, Fontana, 1987.

Dementia and Mental Illness in the Old by E. Murphy, Papermac, 1986.

Don't Say 'Yes' When You Want to Say 'No' by Fensterheim, Herbert and Baer, Futura Publications, (1975).

The Loneliness of the Dying by N. Elias, Blackwell, 1985.

Your Perfect Right: Guide to Assertive Living by R. Alberti, Impact Publications, 1983

Organisations

Age Concern (England) Astral House, 1268 London Road, London SW16 4ER (081–679 8000).

Age Concern (Northern Ireland) 3 Lower Crescent, Belfast BT7 1NR (0232 245729).

Age Concern (Scotland) 54A Fountainbridge, Edinburgh EH3 9PT (031 228 5656).

Age Concern (Wales) 4th floor, 1 Cathedral Road, Cardiff CF1 9SD (0222 371566).

Carers National Association 29 Chilworth Mews, London W2 3RG (071–724 7776).

Support for Relatives of the Elderly Mentally Infirm SREMI Office, Peggy Dodds Centre, 531 Wells Way, Bath BA2 5SW (0225 835520).

Age Care Australia 509 Boundary Road, Toowoomba, QLD 4350, Australia ((008) 800 632).

The Aged Services Association of NSW & ACT Inc Murray Centre, Burwood Road, Burwood, NSW 2134, Australia ((02) 745 2999).

Alzheimer's Association (Australia) Wicks Road, North Ryde, NSW 2113, Australia ((02) 878 4466).

Alzheimer's Association of NSW PO Box 139, Ryde, NSW 2112, Australia ((02) 805 900).

CHAPTER 13

Useful Books

The Disordered Mind: What We Know About Schizophrenia by P. O'Brien, Spectrum, 1978.
Families Helping Families: Living with Schizophrenia by N. Dearth, B. Labenski, M. Mott, L. Pellegrini, Norton, 1984.
Mental Illness and the Law by T. Whitehead, Blackwell, 1983.
Not in our Genes by S. Rose, L. J. Kamin and R. C. Lewontin, Penguin Books, 1984.
The Politics of Experience by R. D. Laing, Penguin Books, 1967.
Schizophrenia and Human Value by P. Barham, Blackwell, 1986.

Personal Accounts

Schizophrenia From Within Edited by J. Wing, The National Schizophrenia Fellowship (this still may be out of print, but your library can order it).

Organisations

National Schizophrenia Fellowship 28 Castle Street, Kingston-upon-Thames, Surrey KT1 1SS (081–547 3937).
Schizophrenia Fellowship of NSW PO Box 111, North Ryde, NSW 2113, Australia ((02) 878 2053).

CHAPTER 14

Useful Books

Many of those listed for Chapter 13 will be useful. In addition: *Images of Destruction* by D. Wigoder, Routledge and Kegan Paul, 1987.

Organisations

The Manic Depression Fellowship Limited 13 Rosslyn Road, Twickenham TW1 2AR (081–892 2811).

Index

229

Index

Piatkus Books

If you are interested in health, recovery and personal growth, you may like to read other titles published by Piatkus.

Recovery

Adult Children of Divorce: How to achieve happier relationships Dr Edward W. Beal and Gloria Hochman (Foreword by Zelda West-Meads of *RELATE*)

At My Father's Wedding: Reclaiming our true masculinity John Lee

Children of Alcoholics: How a parent's drinking can affect your life David Stafford

The Chosen Child Syndrome: What to do when a parent's love rules your life Dr Patricia Love and Jo Robinson

Codependents' Guide to the Twelve Steps: How to understand and follow a recovery programme Melody Beattie

Codependency: How to break free and live your own life David Stafford and Liz Hodgkinson

Don't Call it Love: Recovery from sexual addition Dr Patrick Carnes

Homecoming: Reclaiming and championing your inner child John Bradshaw

Obsessive Love: How to free your emotions and live again Liz Hodgkinson

When Food is Love: Exploring the relationship between eating and intimacy Geneen Roth

Health

Acupressure: How to cure ailments the natural way Michael Reed Gach

The Alexander Technique: How it can help you Liz Hodgkinson

Aromatherapy: The encyclopedia of plants and oils and how they help you Danièle Ryman

Arthritis Relief at Your Fingertips: How to use acupressure massage to ease your aches and pains Michael Reed Gach

The Encyclopedia of Alternative Health Care: The complete guide to choices in healing Kristin Olsen

Herbal Remedies: The complete guide to natural healing Jill Nice

Hypnosis Regression Therapy: How reliving early experiences can improve your life Ursula Markham

Increase Your Energy: Regain your zest for life the natural way Louis Proto

Infertility: Modern treatments and the issues they raise Maggie Jones

Nervous Breakdown: What is it? What causes it? Who will help? Jenny Cozens

Psycho-Regression: A new system for healing and personal growth   Dr Francesca Rossetti

The Reflexology Handbook: A complete guide   Laura Norman and Thomas Cowan

Self-Healing: How to use your mind to heal your body   Louis Proto

The Shiatsu Workbook: A beginners' guide   Nigel Dawes

Spiritual Healing: All you need to know   Liz Hodgkinson

Super Health: How to control your body's natural defences   Christian H. Godefroy

Super Massage: Simple techniques for instant relaxation   Gordon Inkeles

The Three Minute Meditator   David Harp

Women's Cancers: The treatment options   Donna Dawson

Personal Growth

Be Your Own Best Friend: How to achieve greater self-esteem and happiness   Louis Proto

Care of the Soul: How to add depth and meaning to your everyday life   Thomas Moore

Colour Your Life: Discover your true personality through colour   Howard and Dorothy Sun

Creating Abundance: How to bring wealth and fulfilment into your life   Andrew Ferguson

Dare to Connect: How to create confidence, trust and loving relationships   Susan Jeffers

Fire in the Belly: On being a man   Sam Keen

Living Magically: A new vision of reality   Gill Edwards

The Passion Paradox: What to do when one person loves more than the other   Dr Dean C. Delis with Cassandra Phillips

Protect Yourself: How to be safe on the streets, in the home, at work, when travelling   Jessica Davies

The Power of Gems and Crystals: How they can transform your life   Soozi Holbeche

The Power of Your Dreams   Soozi Holbeche

The Right to be Yourself: How to be assertive and make changes in your life   Tobe Aleksander

For a free brochure with further information on our range of titles, please write to:

Piatkus Books
Freepost 7 (WD 4505)
London W1E 4EZ

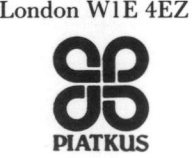

PIATKUS